TIMELINE HISTORY OF LAPAROSCOPY & HERNIA SURGERY

(FOR POSTGRADUATES AND SURGEONS)

Dr. T. Varun Raju

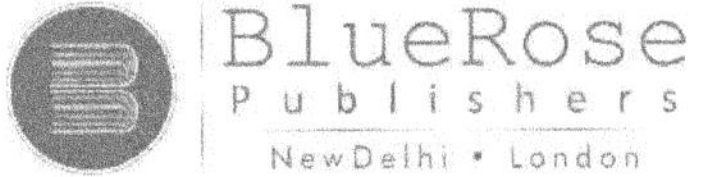

First Published in November 2021

ISBN: 978-93-5472-428-2

BLUEROSE PUBLISHERS

www.bluerosepublishers.com

info@bluerosepublishers.com

+91 8882 898 898

Cover Design:

Geetika

Typographic Design:

Namrata Saini

Distributed by: BlueRose, Amazon, Flipkart, Shopclues

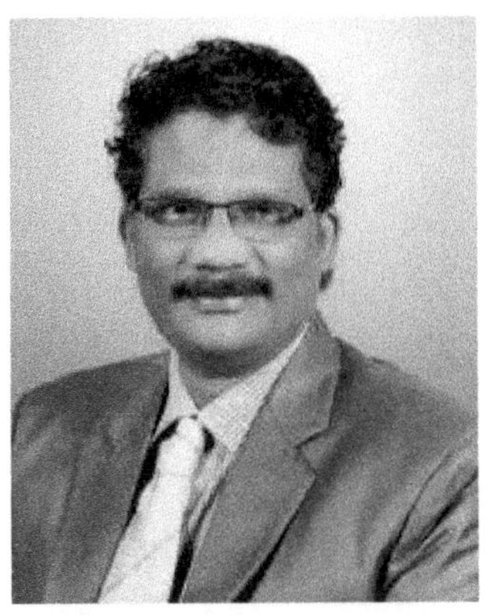

Dr.T.Varun Raju

M.B.B.S, D.N.B (Surgery), FMAS, FIAGS, FALS
(Fellowship in Advanced Laparoscopic Surgery)

Founder and Director TVR Laparoscopy Center & Visiting Consultant Pace Hospitals, Hyderabad

Formery a Teacher D.N.B Postgraduation program (General Surgery), Durgabai – Deshmukh Hospital & Research Center,Hyderabad and H.O.D Minimal Access Surgery, General Surgery,OMNI Hospitals

Dedicated to,

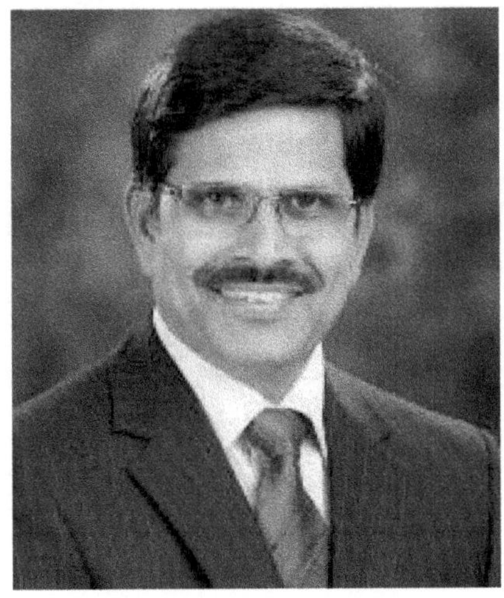

DR. C. PALANIVELU

MS, MCh, DNB, FACS, FRCS (Hon) Edin.

Chairman – GEM Hospital and Research Centre

Professor & Director – Institute of Gastroenterology & Minimal Access Surgery

Coimbattore, Chennai, India.

"A World renowned Surgical Gastro Enterologist, father of Laparoscopic Surgery in India with vast counts of peak positions in the field of minimal access surgery and a very humble teacher to the teachers all over the world"

Foreword

Understanding the history of the development of surgery is not just an exercise in theory. It is a critical analysis of the progressive transformation of the procedure, the initial successes, the debacles, deficiencies, the modifications, and the revolutionary breakthroughs all these steps in the evolutionary cycle of a procedure help us understand the how and why of what we do today. For keen surgical students, a deeper understanding of this process helps him/her become a more complete surgeon overall in terms of procedure selection and patient outcomes. The field of herniology has been one such area of modern medicine that has undergone vast and constant changes, especially in the past half a century. The wide variety of hernias hold varied challenges-some with regards to high failure rates of treatment and some in the areas of faster recovery and better long-term quality of life for these patients. Surgeon scientists over the years have come up with innovative solutions for these challenges. From the open era to the laparoscopic era and now the age of robotics, E-TEP, and abdominal wall reconstruction the field of herniology beautifully illustrates how surgical scientists have risen to the various challenges in delivering improved outcomes in health care and who could be a surgeon better placed to take us through this journey than Dr. Varun Raju. I have known Varun for about a decade now. He is a multi-talented individual with eclectic skills in classical music (he has published several books), singing, painting, digital artistry and publishing in addition of course to being an excellent laparoscopic surgeon,worked along with me in the department of surgical gastro enterology for three years.His passion in the field of herniology and laparoscopic surgery is unmatched. In his 20 odd years as a practicing surgeon, he has made this journey from the open to laparoscopic and E-tep era as a keen updating surgeon of hernia surgery and abdominal wall reconstruction.With his consummate passion, excellent writing skills, and mastery of the craft of hernia surgery he is best placed to guide us through this incredible surgical voyage.

This story telling kind of an interesting history book by Varun is a must-read for not just the eager young surgeon but also the experienced surgical practitioner if he/ she wish to be a more complete surgeon and expert in the field of herniology.

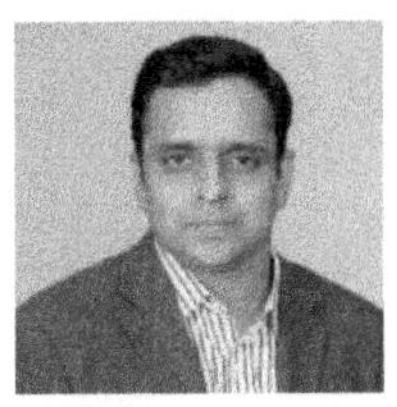

Dr.R.Phani Krshna

M.S (JIPMER), MRCS (EDIN), M.Ch (SGPGI), HPB Oncology Fellowship (Japan),

Liver transplant Fellowship (UK), Senior Surgical Gastro enterologist and Liver transplant surgeon.

Director, PACE Hospitals, Hitech-City Hyderabad, Telangana

Preface

The earliest reference to laparoscopy dates to Biblical history, where Ezekiel wrote, "For the king of Babylon stood at the parting of the way, at the head of the two ways, to use divination: He made his arrows bright, he consulted with images, he looked in the liver (Ezekiel 21:21)."The history of modern endoscopy is relatively young, dating back no more than approximately 130 years ago.This book "Time line history of laparoscopy and hernia surgery (THLH) "is mainly intended to compile the events happened in the past till to the recent times for the development of minimally invasive /Laparoscopic surgery and hernia.The subject is devided in to few chapters according to the time line development milestones found in the reference books, papers and the standard internet data.. The contributors of the history are searched with an aim to find out their original photos with due respect and mentioning the source names. The development of laparoscopy, endoscopy and the hernia surgery are mainly focussed because the aim of this book is unique to enlighten the history in an interesting fashion to the readers. References are given at the end of each chapter and source of the pictures and illustrations are mentioned along with it. I hope this book will be useful to all the post graduate students or surgeons in general surgery and the students learning the minimal access surgery and endoscopy. I am sure this book will be helpful as a guide and a reference book to them during the course of learning surgery or in their surgical practice. I hope this book will be further developed and updated in the future by adding minute details of the development of each invention and the stories behind the struggle of all the laparoscopic /endoscopic instruments or devices and Iam sure that would be more interesting and inspiring to all the future generation surgeons.

Dr.Varun Raju.Thirumalagiri

(Author)

Special appreciation Words

Congratulations, dear Dr.T.Varun Raju.

History of evolution of "The thought of visualising the interior of the Human body, with mechanical means"; Endo/Laparoscopy, with its difficulties, implications, advantages and advancements is well brought out as a time line.

Its role in evolution of Herniae and abdominal wall reconstruction is well presented.My compliments for this great effort. Wishing you all the best.

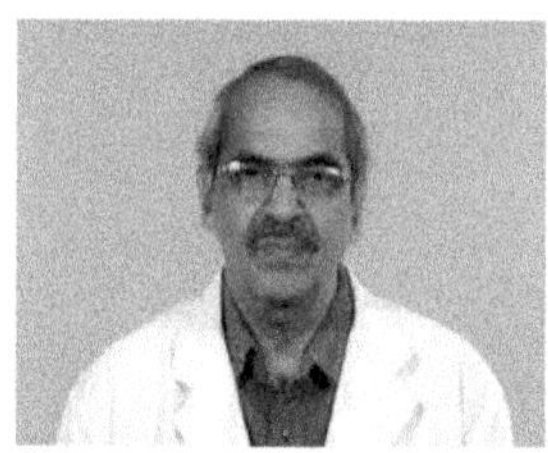

Prof. A .Yadagiri Chary

M.S (General Surgery), Formerly Assistant Professor of Surgery

Gandhi Medical College and Dean of Dr. VRK Women's Medical College, Shadan Institute of Medical Sciences, Hyderabad, Telangana.

Acknowledgements

My thanks list are many of mentors and colleagues in laparoscopic surgery and G.I surgery Dr.B.Narsaiah sir,Ex M.P,Telangana state,Dr.G.suresh Chandra Hari sir, Dr.P.R.K Prasad sir,Dr.Laxman Shastri sir,Dr.L.Sridhar sir,Dr.Vinay sir,Dr.G.V Rao sir,Dr.Ramana BalaSubrahmanyam sir,DR.D.V.L Narayana Rao sir and Dr.Ravula.PaniKrishna.

My special thanks to critics and teachers who inspired, helped and brought out the best in me, Dr.R.S Satwalekar sir, Dr.A.Y.Chary sir, Dr.Beerappa sir, Dr.P.Raghu Ram sir, Dr.Subramanyeshwar rao sir, Dr.G.V .Sudhakar sir Dr.Sri rami raddy sir and Dr.Bhanumathi madam.

I also thank those who have helped me in this book for motivating in many angles Dr.Vamshi ,Dr.Varada Chary for helping me the literature and reference books selection.I also thank L.G.S (Learning General Surgery) a, Telegram group for letting me to download the E-Text books on the subject history of "Laparoscopic surgery,hernia and Abdominal wall reconstruction".

I thank my wife T.Usha Devi, Mother T.Ramulamma and with the guidance of my late father Thirumalagiri Ramulu B.A, B.Ed (retired schools inspector), my sisters and brother for the moral support to finish this important task.

I thank Dr.Palanivelu sir for accepting my request to dedicate my work to him and alo Dr.A.Y Chary sir and Dr.R.Phani Krishna for the priceless appreciative forewords.

Blue Rose publishers Director Mr.Syed Arshad and my project manager Bhanu priya you guys helped me in the production and marketing of this essential book to all the practicing laparoscopic surgeons all over the world.

I cannot end this list without thanking the esteemed readers of the book who keep sending their honest opinions, feedback, suggestions, critical comments etc.Thank you for your kind support and encouragement.

Dr.T.Varun Raju

Director and Chief advanced Laparoscopic,General,G.I &Bariatric Surgeon

T.V.R Laparoscopy Center, Hyderabd.

Contents

1. Introduction

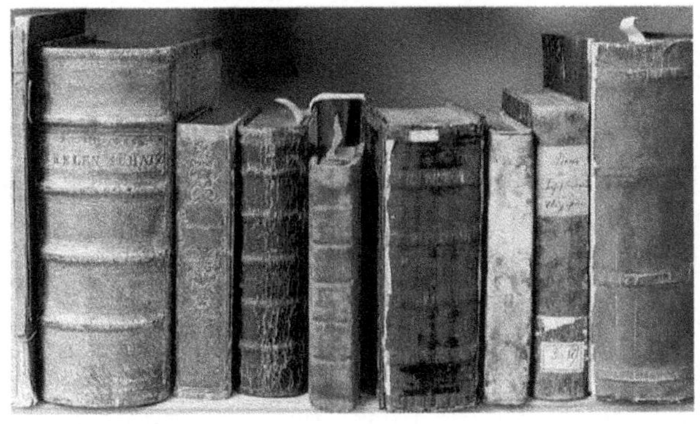

George Moritz Ebers (1837–98), a professor of Egyptology at the University of Berlin, purchased an ancient papyrus while traveling in Egypt in 1873. The papyrus contained a collection of older works dating back to 3000–2500 BC. Ebers prepared a partial translation of the papyrus in 1875, which was later completed by Bendix Ebbell, a Norwegian physician. Ebbell's study of the papyrus suggested that the ancient Egyptians had attained a high level of surgical skill and had developed procedures for hernia and aneurysm management.2 interestingly, then, in the first preserved written record of medical practice, the paradigm for hernia management included surgical intervention. Surgical intervention for hernia, and almost any other disease, was mercifully rare before the modern era. Without anesthesia, operative pain was real and fearsome. In addition, infection almost inevitably followed a surgical procedure and frequently was life-ending. Because of this, the religious proscriptions against human dissection, and technological immaturity, progress in the surgical sciences stagnated. The discovery of anesthesia and the development of antiseptic methods in the mid-nineteenth century revolutionized the practice of surgery. Operative intervention without the twin specters of agonizing operative pain and postoperative infection became possible, and the abdominal cavity no longer remained terra incognita. Along with that for many other diseases, the paradigm for hernia changed

By the end of the 20th century, the old adage 'big surgeon, big incision' had lost its currency: in the future, the small incisions of multiple portal laparoscopic surgery *may* be replaced by single incision laparoscopic surgery (SILS) and in some cases by natural orifice transluminal endoscopic surgery (NOTES), which leaves no external scar.(Moris et al. 2012; Antoniou et al. 2015; Porzionato et al. 2015).

From the ancient times, the four obstacles of the endocscopy were as follows.

1. Creating or expanding entrances to the interior body.

2. Safely delivering enough light in to the interior space.

3. Transmitting a clear and magnified image back to the eye.

4. Expanding the field of vision

It's a well-known fact that, what we are doing our surgical procedures have a strong historical basis. It would be very interesting to know each point of the history if they are chronologically arranged with simple language and narration to the reader. The subject of the history would be interesting to the students and the surgeons if the content is properly searched with the available data from the authoritative sources. It is not that easy to find out the initial point of the development of a surgical instrument in the history because of the evidence gaps, maintenances and preservation in old books which are available in the libraries or in the internet. Any kind of the history will be thrilling and interesting if it's presented to the readers properly according to the time line threading of all the events happened in the past.

I did my way of compilation of the evolutionary historical events of laparoscopic surgery and the technology of auxiliary equipment to support and augment the result of a procedure towards the best results.

I mentioned mostly the historical events happened for the development of laparoscopic/Minimal access surgery in surgical gastroenterology and in hernia surgery because that is my focus basically in this short book presentation.

Laparoscopic hernia surgery is rapidly evolving as a specialized branch because of the advances in technology and equipment with a clear understanding of posterior inguinal regional anatomy, landmarks, and the spaces in the abdominal wall. As the scientific data is accumulating, précised guidelines and recommendations are being evolved through standard hernia societies, collaborations and the associations globally. There has been an impressive and significant development in laparoscopic hernia surgery in the last few decades with sophisticated technical and skill development for learning and performing the procedures in a standardized way of scientific method.

As it's a book of history,I followed the method of vancouer citation of the material for the benefit to the readers because as a writer,I can not change the words or the sentences of the authors who had contributed their original data in the books and the standard journals.I made the book as simple as possible with my best effords and knowledge.

Let us go in to the subject now!

2. Ancient period to 1700 AD

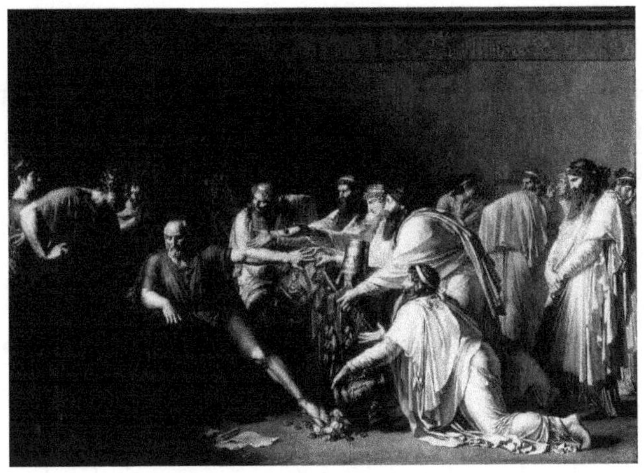

I started my search deep down from the surgery books and in the internet to find out the starting point of the minimal access surgery but realized all the difficulties to standardize the scientific facts and I did my best by initiating the subject as simple as possible now. Let us start very briefly with the historical aspects of exploration of the facts about human anatomy in a chronological way first.

1. Stone age [1] - Cave paintings (about 30,000 years ago) were made depicting simple knowledge of the anatomy of animals.

2. Fifth century B.C.E -Schematic study of anatomy was started by "Alcmaeon & Empedocles" Greek

scientists and performed the first human body dissection[1].Hippocrates was hailed as the "Father of Medicine" and showed the symptoms of a disease.Airstotle was hailed as the "Father of Comparative Anatomy and Physiology" and known as being more philosophical than a physician during those days.

3. During 200A.D – Galen knowledge about anatomy greatly improved from his experience by treating different kinds of wounds.He discovered arteries and 7 out of 12 cranial nerves [2].

4.From 8th Century to 14th Century – The prevailing mood during these periods were not conductive for scientific study and discovery as it centered much in the religious practices and the science became temporarily stagnant[3].

5. During 15th century – Leonardo da Vinci [4] made crude sketches showing various parts of the human body.This period marked the "rebirth" of an empirical study of anatomy. Andreas Vesalius wrote the "De humani corporis fabrica" and was the first accurate description of the interior of the human body .He became the " Father of Modern Anatomy" and William Harvey described the circulation of the blood

6. During 17th Century - Robert Hook's invention of the compound microscope [5] has vastly improved the study of human anatomy.Study of cell structures started from that period.

7. During the 18th century – Dissection of a human body became a recognized punishment and the

dessections were performed on hanged bodies in public.Sir Henry Gray [6] published his book "Anatomy Descriptive and Surgical "a book that revealed the depths of Human anatomy to the world.At present his book which is more commonly known as "Gray's Anatomy" is still the basis for most medical students

8. During the early 19th Century - The study of anatomy improved with the advancement of histology and developmental biology.The idea of "Anatomy theatre 'arose [7].All were permitted the observation of dissections *performed there except the women*

9.20th Century – Is considered as the modern practice of surgery .The limits of previous obstacles are being taken out by the development of the technology and innovations for a surgical procedure by a process of continuous updated attitude of a surgeon. It will go ahead further with no doubts in the future time.

Enthusiasm was the continuous driving force to know about the interiors of a human body as the external anatomical dissections were done with précised descriptions and inventions of the organs.

At the ouset the history of laparoscopy may be divided in to

1. Ancient Egypt

2. Ancient China

3. Ancient India

4. Ancient Greek and Rome

5. Middle East - Al-Quasim,Al-Haytham,Ibn Sina - Establishes world's earliest endoscopic techniques.

The ability to look within a body cavity [8] in a living patient was a long held dream in medicine. Until the early 19th century the diagnosis of a patient's malady, unless it was visible or easily palpated, was a secret that the body yielded only at surgery or autopsy, the former procedure associated with death just a little less than the latter.

In fact, endoscopic-like tools and practices have been discovered in Egypt as far back as 1700-1600 BCE in a text called the Edwin Smith Papyrus [9]. This text describes endoscopic procedures and the rudimentary tools used for them but more impressively the text cites an older document from 2640 BCE [9] making it some of the earliest known writings about endoscopy.

A manuscript discovered by the American Egyptologist Edwin Smith referred to as Edwin Smith Papyrus, allowed us to elucidate some rudimentary endoscopic techniques dating from **2640 BC** (Fig - 01). This is the oldest known document dealing with surgery. It was written, or more likely recopied, around **1500**. The first doctors who appeared in Rome were Greeks, captured and brought as prisoners of war. Roman specimens have been found to have anal and vaginal speculum, which proves that they are examining the size and state of the internal organs accessible by the natural orifices and were able to thus make diagnoses and to practice interventions.

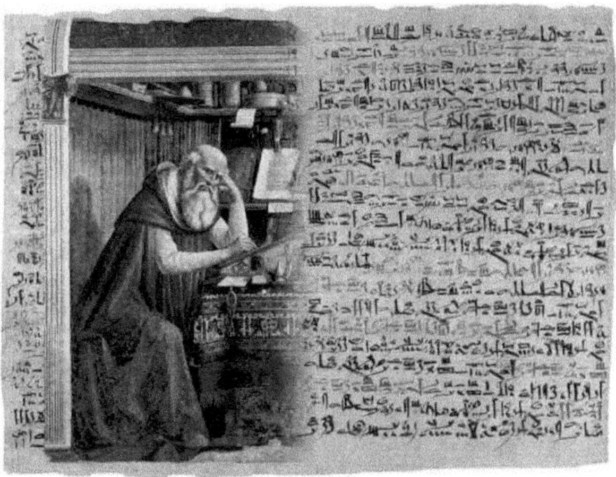

Fig -01 Edwin Smith Papyrus

Vaginal specula

Among the most complex instruments used by Roman and Greek physicians. Most of the vaginal specula discovered consist of a screw device with 2 (sometimes 3 or 4) valves which, when turned, forces a cross-bar to push the blades outwards.

Through recommended by Graeco-Roman physicians who specialize in the field of gynecology and obstetrics, the first author who makes mention of this would be Soranus of Ephesus, for its specific use for vaginal disorders [10].

The concept of minimally invasive surgery has been present since a very long period and started with the advent of endoscopy of the rectum, vagina, ear, and nose. The word Laparoscopy was derived from ancient Greek "λαπάρα"- lapara, meaning: flank" and, σκοπέω – Skopeo, meaning "to see". Those who would like to know the History of Laparoscopic Surgery must look at the earliest stages of development of Endoscopy and Endoscopy traces its origins to two of the easiest access points of the human body; the rectum and the vagina.

The oldest description of an endoscopic examination comes from the Kos School of Hippocrates (Fig- 02) in Greece (**460 – 375 BC**) which created rectal speculum an instrument mentioned by him, which allowed physicians to examine the rectal cavity of a patient.[11]

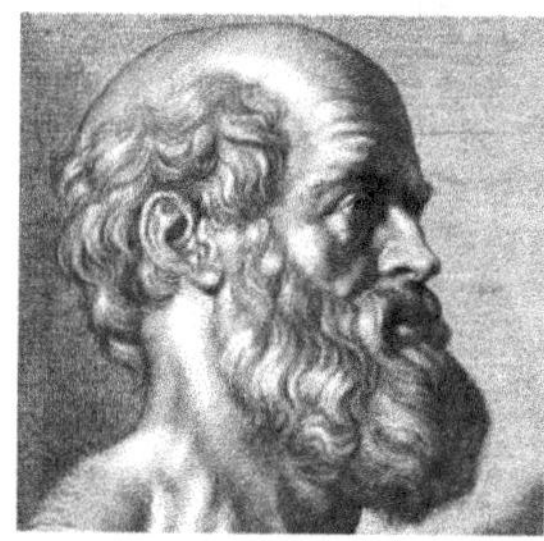

Fig- 02 Hippocrates

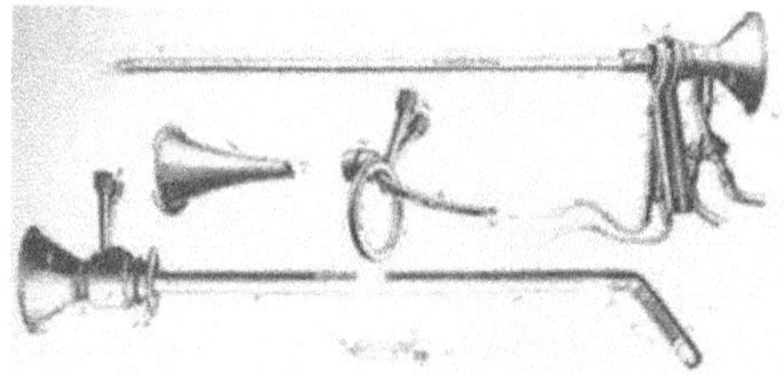

Fig –03 Endoscopic instruments

As well, Hippocrates insisted on finding a natural, rather than supernatural, understanding of disease. With his great skill in observation and analysis, Hippocrates was able to achieve an understanding of disease pathologies that were often previously attributed to supernatural inflictions. Most notably too, Hippocrates was one of the greatest advocates for minimally invasive medicine. Recognizing the value of a minimalist approach, he stressed that physicians, instead of trying to interfere with the body's own healing powers, should instead seek to restore harmony by prescribing diet, rest, exercise and even music as therapy. He also explored the realm of endoscope technology found in his book The Art of Medicine in 400BC [9].

His work describes in great detail how a speculum can be used to visually examine the rectum in section 5 titled On Hemorrhoids [9] .

Just after the Egyptians and Greeks, the Romans also began utilizing endoscopic technique and instruments in the first century CE [12]. Surgical tools have been unearthed in the volcanic ruins of Pompeii most spectacular of which are the specula and urinary catheters, which allowed a diseased body to be cured without an open procedure [13] .

An analogous instrument used for the rectum, vagina, nose and ear, was found in the ruins of Pompei [14]. The Babylonian Talmund (500 BC) described a similar vaginal speculum: Abulcasis of Cordoba (980 - 1013, according to other authors 936 - 1013)

Many countries and continents have contributed the development of the science by making new instruments to examine the inside parts of the human body with enthusiasm and interest to cure the diseases.The Indians have contributed endoscopic methods which were documented in the book "Shushruta-Samahita"[15]- **600 B.C**. (Fig - 04) some first descriptions of a speculum used for the examinations of the inner ear were also found in these works, in other words, what might be called today otoscopy.(Fig -05)

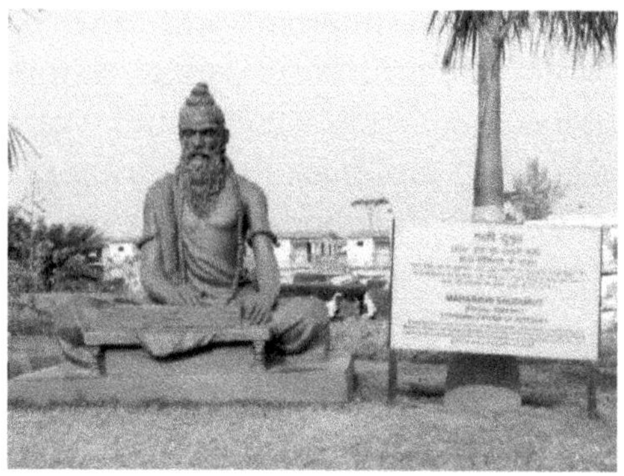

(Fig -4)

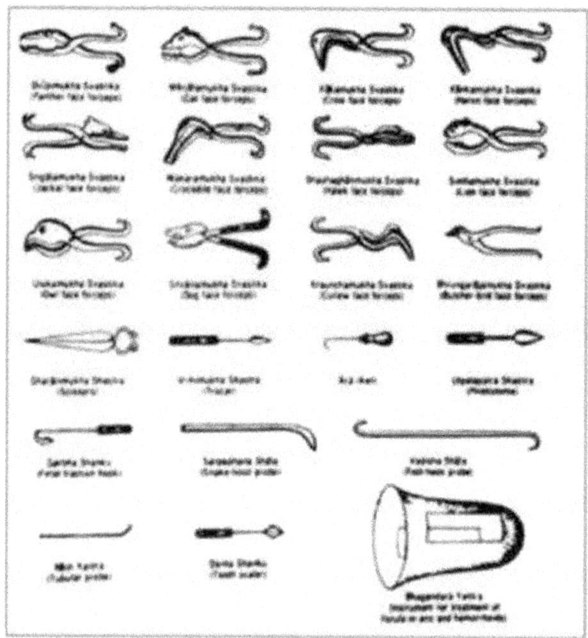

(Fig -5)

According to Sushrutha, endoscopes are the instruments which are categorized under tubular instruments of the main group of blunt instruments [16]. Tubular instruments are of several types and they are used in a variety of situations. They are used for the examination and treatment of diseased spots of external orifices like ear, nose, mouth, vagina and rectum. They have a hollow interior with an opening at one or both ends. Some have one or two openings on the sides as well. Those with openings at both ends are used for inspection of the throat and extraction of foreign bodies from it.

They are also used for aspiration and facilitating surgical operations on external orifices. Shushruta, known today as one of the "fathers of surgery" for his exceptional skill and knowledge. Like the Egyptian Smith's Papyrus and the Chinese Nei-Ching, this Indian treatise also referred back to medical knowledge established as early as 2800 BC.

Later in the 10th century, Albukasim, (Fig - 06) an Arab physician, developed methods of speculum illumination with candlelight and mirrors. Abū al-Qāsim Khalaf ibn al-'Abbās Al-Zahrawi was born and raised in Al-Zahra', a suburb of the town of Qurttoba (Cordova) in Andalucia (now in Spain). He is known in the Western literature as Albucasis, Abulcasis, Bucasis. He was an innovative surgeon who added many original contributions to surgery and medicine.He remained a renowned teacher of surgery through his well-known single, practical and encyclopaedic work Al-Tasrif Li-man 'Ajaza 'An al-Ta'alif.

The history of endoscopy can be dated back to the 10th century when he **(936–1013 AD)** used reflected light to inspect the cervix [14] He described his speculum as "two rods, one lying on the top of the other, which are introduced into the cervix (he probably meant vagina) to expand it with the help of screws".He invented several devices used during surgery, for purposes such as inspection of the interior of the urethra.

By inventing a new instrument, an early form of the lithotrite which he called "Michaab", he was able to crush the stone inside the bladder without the need for a surgical incision.[17]

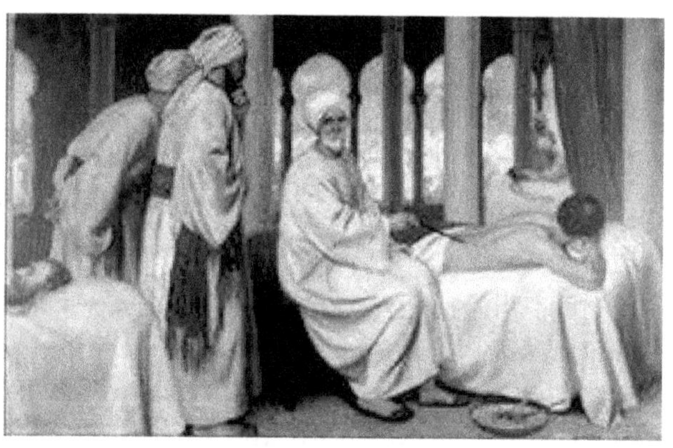

Fig – 06 Albukasim an Arab physician

Regarding the contribution of Chinese physicians in the history of surgery and endoscopy, it was not precisely found by the fact that, due to the religious stigma attached to the practice of surgery, the social position accorded to the surgeon became increasingly lower and thus made a revival of Chinese surgery impossible."[18] Important Chinese contributions include early versions of catheters and understanding of the *camera obscura* phenomenon, knowledge of which would later of course influence the development of integral components of endoscopy. As for the catheter, it has a rich history at least 2000 years old as an integral part of medical practices throughout numerous ancient societies. China's version of a catheter was described as consisting of hollow leaves, referred to in Latin as *allium fistulosum.*

Hua Tuo (c. **140–208**), courtesy name Yuanhua, was a Chinese physician who lived during the late Eastern Han dynasty.[19]This loss to traditional Chinese medicine was irreplaceable. Ilza Veith notes that, "Unfortunately, Hua T'o's works were destroyed; his surgical practices fell into disuse, with the exception of his method of castration, which continued to be practised. Hua Tuo's innovative anaesthetic *mafeisan* (literally "cannabis boiling powder", considered to be the first anesthetic in the world.[20] which was supposedly used on Hua Tuo's patients during surgery, is a long-standing mystery [21]. Almost 2500 years ago, one of China's most famous philosopher's, Mo-tzu (470-391 BC) described what may have been the first accounts of camera obscura principles, which he termed "the locked treasure room" (also "the collecting place").

Visibility, which includes lenses and optics, illumination, and camera technology, also had some of the most difficult hurtles to overcome in comparison to the most basic method of accessing the interior of the body by an incision. Lenses are a relatively modern invention. Optical lenses had been in existence since the early 11th century by the **1683** when a Dutch scientist, Antony van Leeuwenhoek, invented the microscope lens [22]. Leeuwenhoek got the ball rolling and 27 years later the next advancement in optics evolved.

The revolutionary development of the science of the light and it's properties,colours,perception of light and many human physiological aspects have led the history of the practice of medicine in to another level. Since the discovery of fire, people have strived to create better and brighter light sources. The origin of artificial light goes all the way back to **500 BC**, when bamboo pipes carried natural gas from volcanoes to light the streets of ancient China. Later, the Romans lit the front of their homes with oil lanterns and had special servants who tended to these lanterns. In **1417**, the Mayor of London created a law that required all homes have a lantern hung front during the winter.

The European Scientific Revolution between the **1500s–1700s** made a fairly large leap forward, beginning with the year **1500**, a year commonly cited as the starting point for the modern era of scientific history.

In the opening hours of this modern era, one of the first documented attempts to harness artificial light was achieved by the famed though somewhat controversial Italian mathematician-physician named Gerolamo Cardano. (Fig - 07) **(1501-1576)**, whose life work exemplified the Renaissance era of rambunctious intellectualism,. Cardano clearly broke the mold for endoscopy at this time with his invention of a mechanical lamp for examining interior body cavities.

Credit is given to the Frenchman Pierre Borel of Castres (**1620-1689**), the personal physician to King Louis XIV, for inventing the concave mirror that reflects light more intensely and precisely. Borel (Fig – 08) is also considered among the first to apply the microscope to medicine.

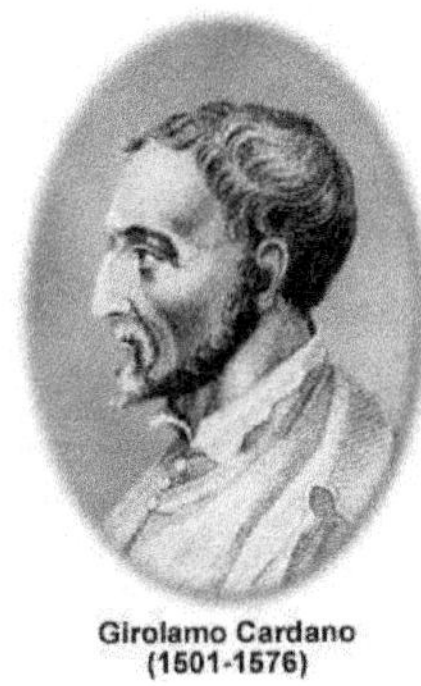

Fig – 07 Gerolamo Cardano (1501-1576)

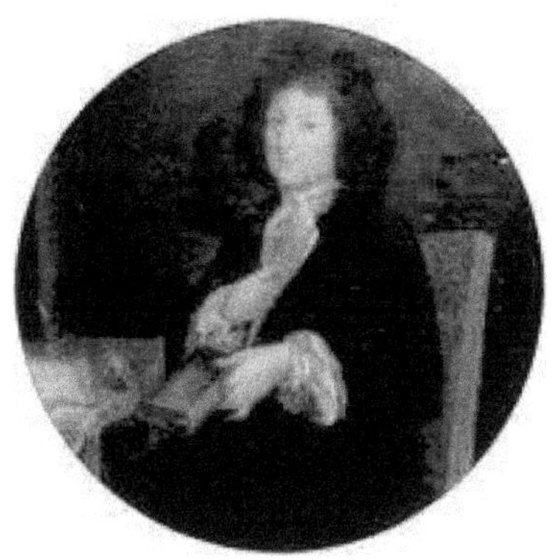

Fig – 08 Pierre Borel of Castres (1620-1689) .
Italian mathematician-physician

The game changing event of laparoscopic surgery, a historical step initiated by Giulio Cesare Aranzi in **1585** (Fig - 09) from Bologna, was the first to use a light source to visualize a cavity in the human body. To achieve this, he tried to illuminate the rectal and vaginal cavities with reflected natural light (focused sunlight) through a flask of water and projected it to visualize the nasal cavity also. [23].

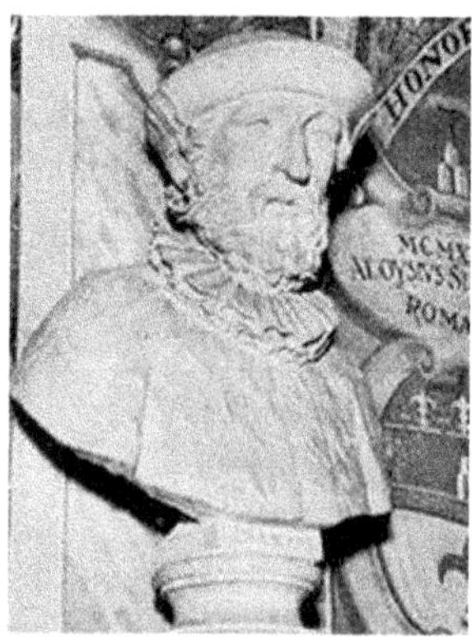

Fig – 09 Giulio Cesare Aranzi (1530 – 1589)

References

1. Carola, Robert. 1992. A Short History of Human Anatomy
2. “Galen.” Famous Scientists. famousscientists.org. 22 Dec. 2014
3. HistoryofAnatomy 2016. http://www.historyworld.net/wrldhis/PlainTextHistories.asp?historyid=aa05
4. “History of anatomy and physiology: The Renaissance and Age of Enlightenment.” World of Anatomy and Physiology, 2007 June 15

5. Robert Hooke - 1635-1703 - Hooke's Microscope
6. Johnson, D. (2016). Introductory Anatomy. Accessed July 20, 2016
7. Cynthia Klestinec - Journal of the History of Medicine and Allied Sciences, *Volume 59, Number 3, July 2004, pp. 375-412*
8. The minimally invasive operations that transformed surgery, Don K. Nakayama, MD, MBA- American college of surgeons,2017.
9. Nezhat, Dr. Camran, and Barbara Page. "ANCIENT TO PRE-MODERN PERIOD." 'History of Endoscopy' Ed. Dr. Paul Alan Wetter. Society of Laproendoscopic Surgeons, 1 Jan. 2005. Web. 16 Mar. 2015.
10. *"Surgical Instruments from Ancient Rome"*. University of Virginia Claude Moore Health Services Library. 2007. *Retrieved 16 September2014*
11. *"Surgical Instruments from Ancient Rome"*. University of Virginia Claude Moore Health Services Library. 2007. *Retrieved 16 September2014*
12. Surgical and Imageguided Technologies. Hoboken, N.J.: John Wiley & Sons Culjat, Martin, Rahul Singh, and Hua Lee. Medical Devices, 2012. 3-9.
13. Culjat, Martin, Rahul Singh, and Hua Lee. Medical Devices Surgical and Imageguided Technologies. Hoboken, N.J.: John Wiley & Sons, 2012. 3-9.
14. Spaner SJ, Warnock GL. A brief history of endoscopy, laparoscopy, and laparoscopic surgery. J Laparoendosc Adv Surg Tech A 1997;7:369-73.
15. Original Article, Sushruta: Ihe Internet Journal of Plastic Surgery Volume Number 2, 2006) plastic Surgeon in 600 B.C. S Saraf, R Parihar.

16. Indian J Surg. 2008 Oct; 70(5): 219–223.

17. Butt, Arthur J. (1956). Etiologic Factors in Renal Lithiasis. Thomas.

18. Veith, Ilza (1966). *Huang Ti Nei Ching Su Wen; The Yellow Emperor's Classic of Internal Medicine*. University of California Press

19. de Crespigny, Rafe (2007). *A biographical dictionary of Later Han to the Three Kingdoms (23–220 AD)*. Leiden: Brill.

20. Cooper, Raymond; Che, Chun-Tao; Mok, Daniel Kam-Wah; Tsang, Charmaine Wing-Yee (2017). Chinese and Botanical Medicines: Traditional Uses and Modern Scientific Approaches. CRC Press. p. 129.

21. Ross, Stewart (2019). The First of Everything: A History of Human Invention, Innovation and Discovery. Michael O'Mara Books. p. 42.

22. Nezhat, Dr. Camran, and Barbara Page. "RENAISSANCE, SCIENTIFIC REVOLUTION, AGE OF ENLIGHTENMENT." 'History of Endoscopy' Ed. Dr. Paul Alan Wetter. Society of Laproendoscopic Surgeons, 1 Jan. 2005. Web. 16 Mar. 2015.

23. Gotz F, Pier A, Schippers E, Schumpelick V. The history of laparoscopy. In: Gotz F, Pier A, Schippers E, Schumpelick V, editors. Color Atlas of Laparoscopic Surgery. New York 1993:3-

3. 1700 to 1865 AD

Intercalarily, with the understanding of anatomy developed in the Renaissance period[1], many medical devices were invented. On the other hand this shows that the importance of medical-based devices is understood and more studies have been initiated to improve them. The emerging different types of diseases have increased the need for medical devices such as trocars. Although the use of trocars is thought to date back thousands of years, they emerged in the early **19th century** and as a result of years of research on trocars, Reginald Southey (Fig -10) an English physician, invented the Southey tube. Thus, trocars have become usable medical devices.

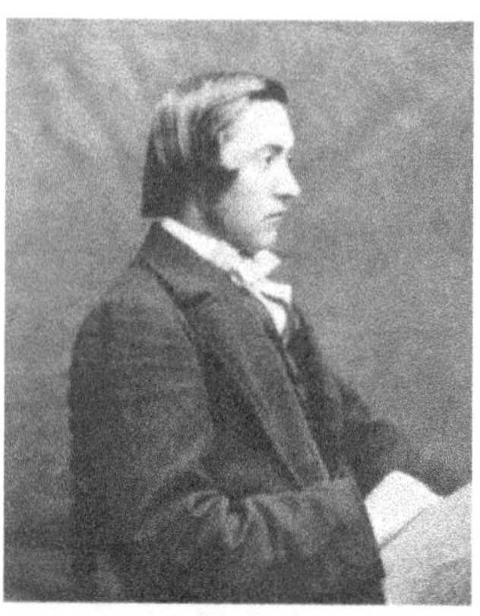

Fig – 10 Reginald Southey (1835 – 1899),

Indeed, as early as **1706**, the term "trocar" was apparently first coined, a word thought to have derived from trochartor troise-quarts, which describes a three-faced instrument consisting of a perforator enclosed in a metal cannula. The term trocar was first used by the British however, it is believed to be derived from French "trois-quarts," (Fig-11) a three-faceted instrument consisting of a cutter in a metal sleeve that was used for withdrawing fluids from a body cavity.

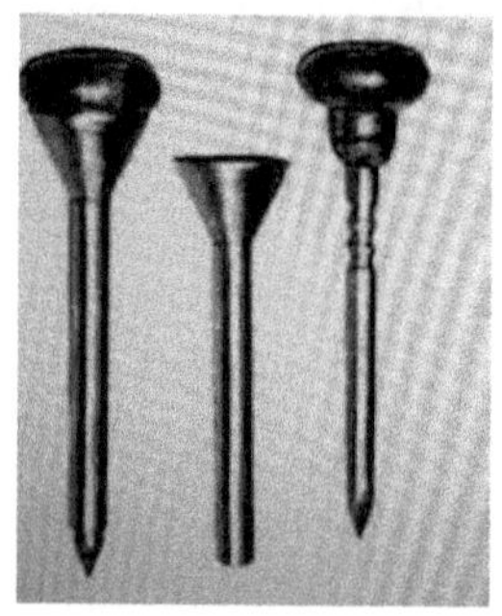

Fig – 11 Trois-quarts

By **1710** there was a leap in optical technology, which was nicely summed up in a textbook called The First

Optical Instruments as Allegorical Depiction by the German author, Johann Michael Conradi.[2] (Fig - 12)

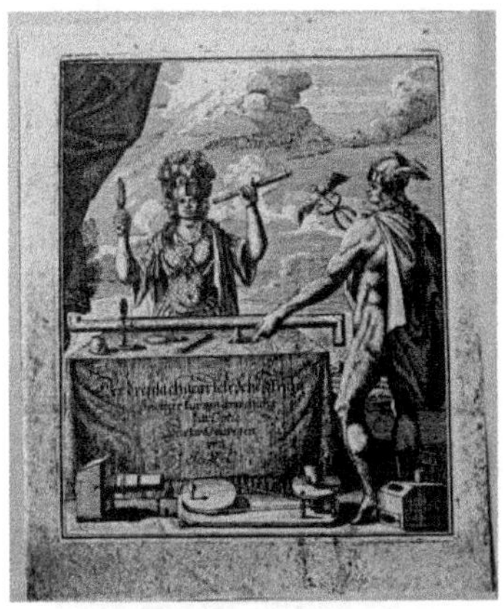

Fig – 12 Johann Michael Conradi

Johann Michael Conradi compiled the textbook on the evolution of optics, cleverly entitled which also included remarks about endoscopy's history. He compiled a textbook on the evolution of optics, cleverly entitled *The First Optical Instruments as Allegorical Depiction*, (Fig -13) which also included remarks about endoscopy's history. Remarkably, Conradi's work provides for an unexpected revelation, for it reveals that almost all elements necessary to make the endoscope viable existed at this very early juncture in time. Using the framework of optical technologies, Conradi outlined the roots of endoscopy and summarized the development of endoscopic technologies from the previous centuries. A number of optical instruments were depicted in fine detail (Fig-14). What is most striking is that, based on these diagrams, one can see that every single part necessary for Bozzini's endoscope was in fact already available. Even many of the parts necessary for Nitze's work were pictured. The full list of items included a prism similar to the one utilized by Trouve and Nitze, magnifying glasses, microscopes, lenses, a lamp case, and a conical mirror (both flat and curved) used for distorting, a feature necessary for future otoscopes and periscopes. Just missing from the list were galvanized wires and electricity, which naturally were not available during this 1710 time frame.

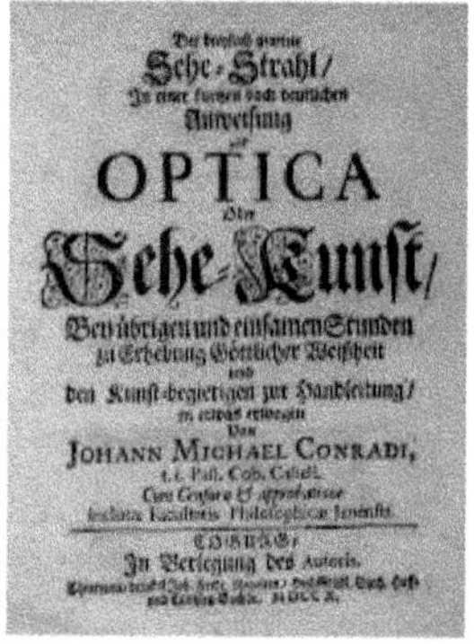

Sehe-Strahl/
Anweisung
OPTICA
Oder
Sehe-Kunst/
Bey übrigen und einsamen Stunden
zu Erhebung Göttlicher Weißheit
und
den Kunst-begierigen zur Handleitung/
Von
JOHANN MICHAEL CONRADI,
In Verlegung des Autoris.

Fig - 13

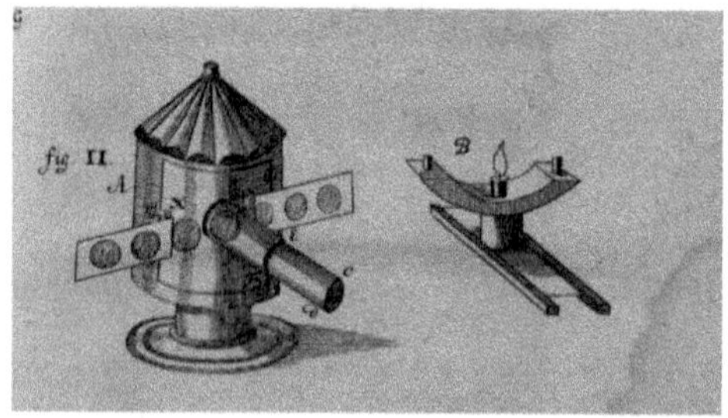

Fig – 14

Conradi's Optical Instruments

One has to look at the early 1800s in order to discover the next leap ahead. In the early 19th century, Philip

Bozzini **(1773–1809)**(Fig - 15) Philip Bozzini an Obstetrician from Frankfurt, Germany was the first to design and build a self-contained instrument with light source and mechanics to illuminate the interior cavities and spaces of the living body with reflected light to examine the urethra and bladder.. He utilized the centrally bored mirror for his cystoscope.

He called this device the "Lichtleiter" [3](Fig - 16) or "light conductor". In **1806**, a leather-lined box that held a candle interposed in the sightline between the examiner's eye and a speculum wedged into the urethra or vagina to inspect for signs of venereal disease, urethral strictures, and bladder stones. Originally, the lichleiter was designed mostly with obstetric and gynecologic inspections in mind, since Bozzini's initial training was in this field. And it appears that the most success with the lichleiter was in examining female patients. In this field, Bozzini became especially frustrated that only blind palpation was available as a means of examination. He demonstrated this to the Medical Faculty in Vienna, which not only rejected this sort of "magical lantern", but also censured Bozzini for his "morbid curiosity" [4]. In fact, a common saying during his time was that "the eye of the obstetrician should be located in his fingertips." Yet, this was a view Bozzini did not share in the least. Bozzini is quoted as stating that such inspections relied "merely on good luck and chance." He firmly believed that such games of chance could finally be ended by using his device.

He first presented his idea to the public in **1804** and officially on February 7, **1805**. In July of 1806, the instrument was demonstrated at a scientific session in

Frankfurt. He demonstrated this to the Medical Faculty in Vienna, which not only rejected this sort of "magical lantern", but also censured Bozzini for his "morbid curiosity". However, the idea did not go unnoticed: during the same year R. Fisher in the United States and the following year M. Segales in France carried out vaginal examinations using reflected light applying Bozzini's idea.He made the Beginning of Early Modern Endoscopy **1806.**

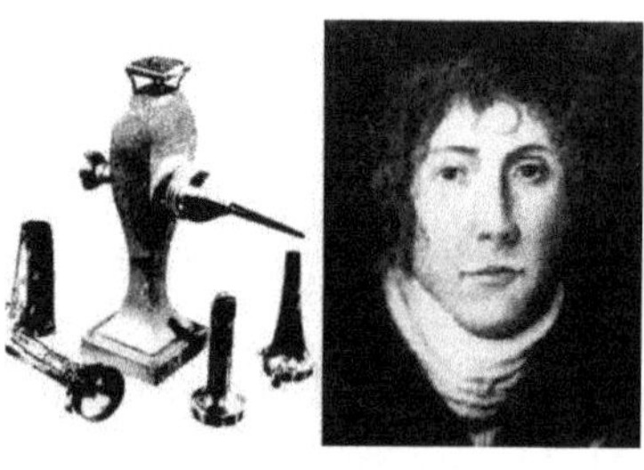

Fig – 15 Philip Bozzini

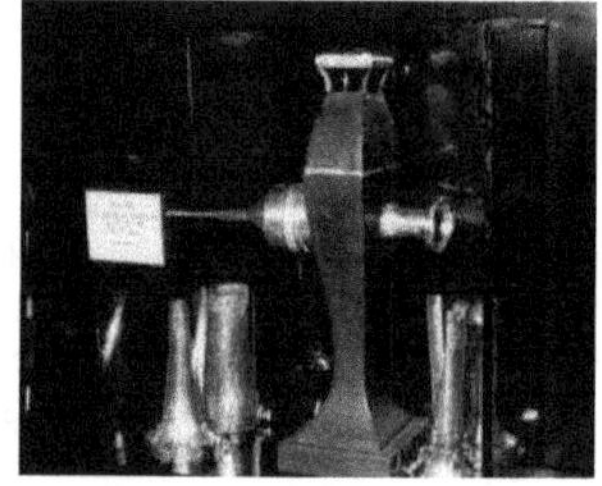

Fig – 16 Lichtleiter

In reviewing the history, it seems Bozzini faced at least three main types of obstacles: 1) technical difficulties, 2) time constraints, and 3) resistance and rivalry from colleagues. The other immediately observable setback relates to the untimely and unfortunate demise of Bozzini himself, who succumbed to typhoid fever on April 4, 1809, just about a month before his 36th birthday.

Curiously too, the amazing fact that **Levret** was possibly the first ever to have performed a therapeutic endoscopic procedure using reflected light other than sunlight also seems to have slipped past the world's notice.

Refereences

1. Missori, Paolo; Brunetto, Giacoma M.; Domenicucci, Maurizio (7 February 2012). "Origin of the Cannula for Tracheotomy During the Middle Ages and Renaissance". *World Journal of Surgery*. **36** (4): 928–934.

2. Nezhat, Dr. Camran, and Barbara Page. "HOVERING ON THE BRINK OF MODERNITY." 'History of Endoscopy' Ed. Dr. Paul Alan Wetter. Society of Laproendoscopic Surgeons, 1 Jan. 2005.

3. Bozzini PH. Lichtleiter, eine Erfindung zur Anschauung innerer Theile und Krankheiten nebst der Abbildung. J Practis Arzneyk Wunderarzneyk. 1806;**24**:107–124

4. Spaner SJ, Warnock GL. A brief history of endoscopy, laparoscopy, and laparoscopic surgery. J Laparoendosc Adv Surg Tech A 1997;7:369-73.

4. 1865 AD to World war II

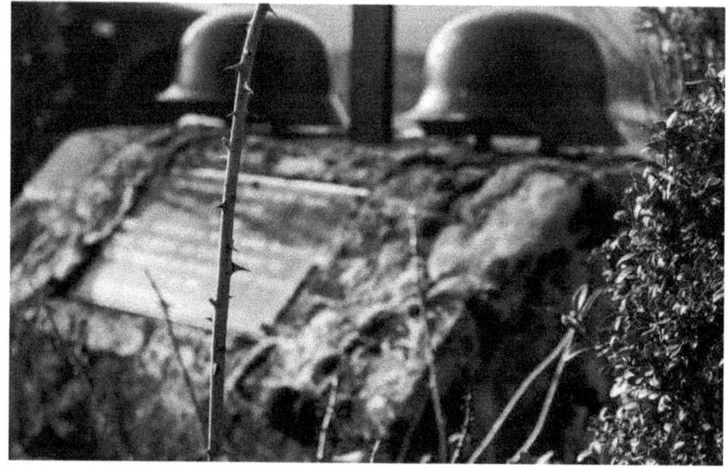

Antonin Desormeaux of Paris (Fig- 17) presented the first "modern" cystoscope to the Academy of Medicine in Paris. He presented the first description of a cystoscope to the Academy of Medicine in Paris in 1855, [1,2] has been described as the "Father of Endoscopy" for the discoveries and technology that grew out of his work.[3] The examination carried out with this instrument is considered the first true endoscopy in history. In **1883** he replaced the candle with an alcohol and turpentine-burning lamp. The light was brighter but the contraption became dangerously hot, a problem in a device held so close to the patient's perineum and the examiner's face. Desormeaux replaced Bozzini's unwieldy speculums with a long tube, creating the first true cystoscope (Fig - 18). His other lasting contribution was the name of his apparatus, which he called “l’endoscopie.”. In **1865, Sir Francis Richard Cruise of Dublin** was the first to explore a body cavity, the empyema cavity in the thorax of an 11-year-old girl, using a cystoscope of Desormeaux’s design that he modified to produce more light.

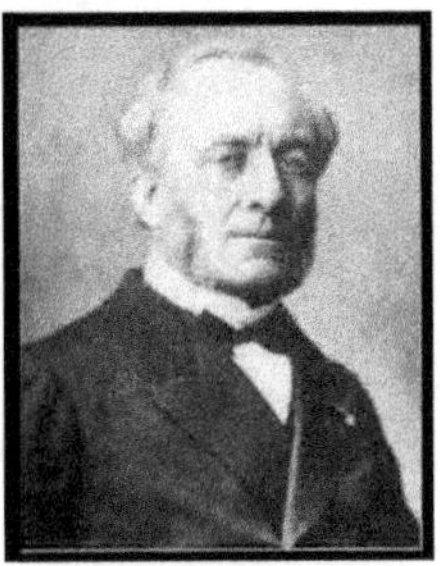

Fig- 17 Antoine Jean Desormeaux (1867)

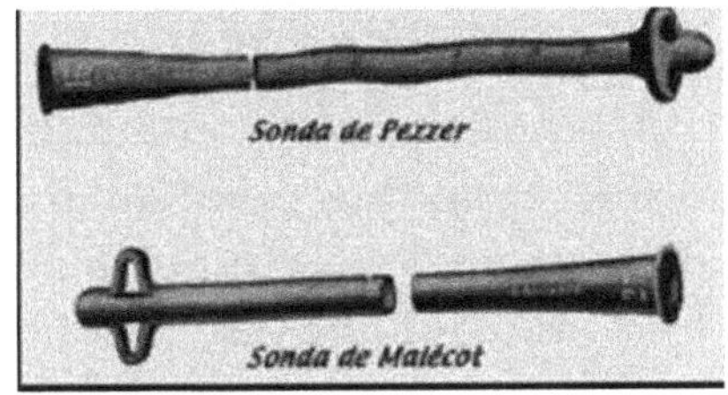

Fig - 18 First true cystoscope

At about the same time, new instrument models were being developed in the United States. The best was an instrument designed in **1860** by Phillip Skinner[4] Wales while he was doing postgraduate study at the University of Pennsylvania. His creation, (Fig – 19) was produced by Horatio Kern, a well-known instrument maker in Philadelphia. Wales' instrument contains a metal shaft, again with a very acute beak, but it uses an ophthalmologic mirror to reflect light down the channel. One peers through the center hole to look into the bladder. It was elegant, light, and relatively easy to use.

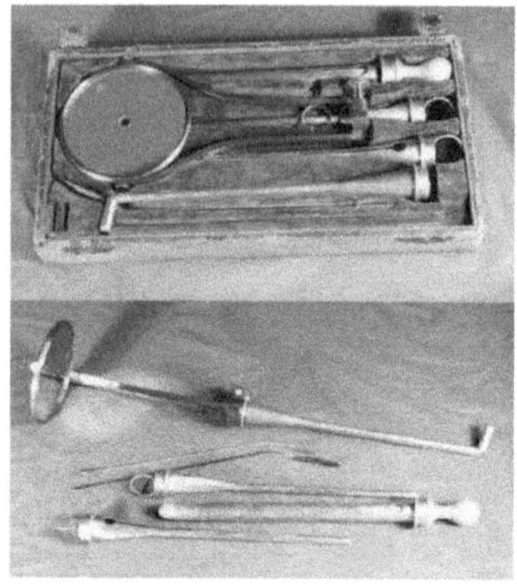

Fig 19 – Philip Skinner's Cystoscope.

In **1867** a dentist from Breslau, Karl Ludwig von Bruck created the first instrument with an internal light. This invention became a turning point in the History of Endoscopy: many practitioners attempted to insert the light bulb into the endoscopes, causing numerous burns.

"whether perhaps bolder species of a distant future will attempt, in such cases through gastrotomy, creation of a gastric fistula and dilatation of the stricture with a knife or probe, to achieve radical successes ... who dares today to decide this question? One must fear being softly or loudly ridiculed for just posing it" [5] .

In **1870** Adolph Kussmaul (Fig – 20) performed esophagoscopy using a rigid tube with mirrors: he had the idea while watching a sword swallowing show! (Fig – 21) he first used instrument down the esophagus and into his guinea pig like sword swallower. Kussmaul carefully observed the sword swallower, being especially interested in the way he positioned his head for the passage of the long, straight sword, and then decided to examine him with the Desormeaux endoscope. For this purpose he had a local instrument-maker fashion tubes 47 cm long and 13 mm in diameter, one being of round, the other of elliptical section. The tubes were fitted with conical wooden mandarins to facilitate insertion.

The sword-swallower tolerated the long tubes well, but the examination was disappointing because the light was too weak to illuminate a field so far from its source. Also, despite washing out the stomach, fluid constantly collected round the tube and hindered the view. This is probably the first time that acid reflux was observed, and the lack of a suction apparatus must have been a great drawback.

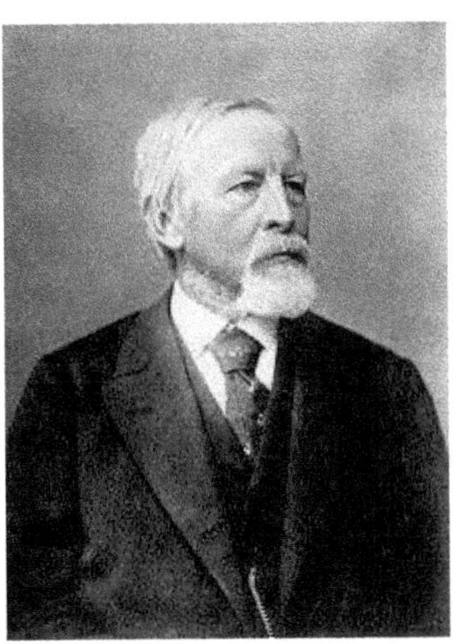

Fig – 20 Adolph Kussmaul

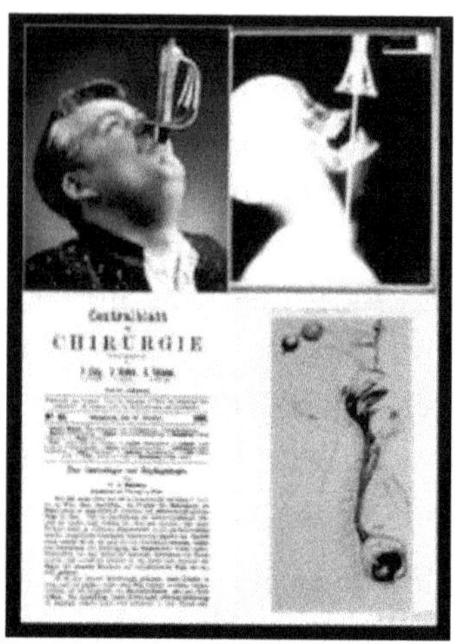

Fig – 21 Sword swallowing show

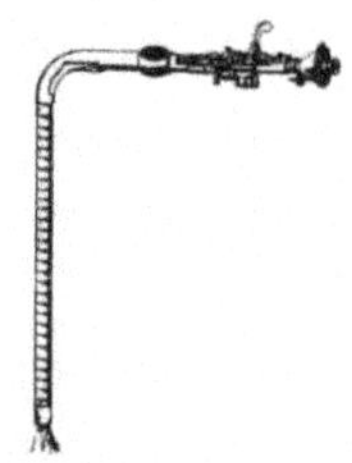

Fig – 22

Flexible or right-angled instruments continued to be designed and used, such as that of Nietze and Leiter in 1881[6] (Fig 22). This complex piece of apparatus deserves mention on account of its optical system, which incorporated primitive distal lighting. As with Mikulicz's instrument, the platinum glow-light employed gave out so much heat that a watercooling system was required, making the apparatus somewhat complicated and cumbersome.

Even as late as 1912 angled instruments were still used. That of Lewisohn illustrates an improved proximal lighting system and a telescopic tube [7].

1876 Maximilian Nitze, (Fig - 23) modified Edison's light bulb invention and created the first optical endoscope with the built-in electrical light bulb as the source of illumination [8]. He Invented the first cystoscope (Nitze–Leiter cystoscope) in 1879 using an electrically heated platinum wire for illumination and created the first electric light bulb for use during urological procedures.Like the Lichtleiter from Bozzini, this instrument was only used for urologic procedures. In **1879**, he improved the cystoscope, adding a platinum wire electric light source and developing the first endoscopic photographs.

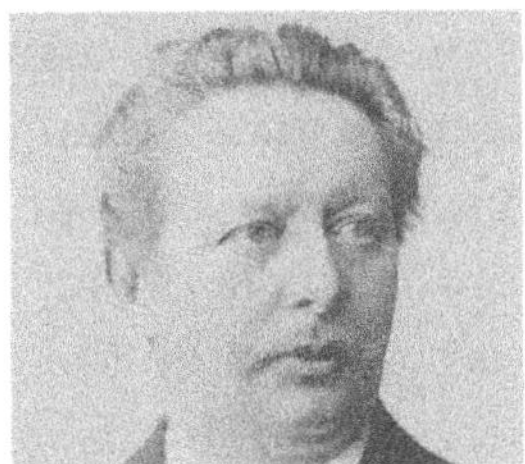

Fig – 23 Maximilian Carl-Friedrich Nitze. (1848 –1906) German urologist.

In October of **1878**, Leiter wrote to Nitze that "the instruments have been finished completely for practical use". Shortly thereafter in October, Leiter himself brought these instruments to Dresden. Nitze was bitterly disappointed, since not a single instrument could be used clinically. Finally, in December 1878, Maximilian Nitze moved to Vienna to personally supervise the further construction of the instruments.

This close cooperation between Nitze and Leiter did prove successful [9].

On 9 May 1879, during a session of the Royal Imperial Society of Physicians in Vienna, the surgeon Leopold von Dittel presented the first cystoscope by Nitze and Leiter, urethroscope and rectoscope on a patient to the medical public.Immediately after this groundbreaking demonstration Max Nitze wrote [10] his treatise "On a new illumination method of the cavities of the human body" which was published in the 26th volume of the *Wiener Medizinische Wochenschrift* in **1879**. The scientific world listened and the international reception was enthusiastic.

Two other pioneers, Czechlasovakian Johann von Mikulicz and Joseph Leiter from Vienna, also paved the way to illumination. But, like many inventors, they developed endoscopy in more than one way. In **1881** the two men improved the current optical system in circulation by incorporating a prism[11]. It should also be noted that they were one of the first to advance tubing technology to be discussed in its respective category. Although Trouve had already introduced prisms into his circle of peers, Mikulicz and Leiter were the first to do so in regard to their own procedures and in combination with their respective illumination and tubing designs[11].

Johannes Freiherr surgeon of Polish-Lithuanian descent born in Bukowina, Romania, constructed the first rigid endoscope in **1880** and was the first to use Edison's light bulb for his gastroscope in practice.

He modified the instrument so that it could be angled by 30 degrees near to its lower third to achieve better visualization. He added a separate channel for air insufflation. In one of the first interventional endoscopic procedures, he pushed a large swallowed bone from the esophagus into the stomach, thus avoiding surgery - surgeon in the evolution of flexible endoscopy[12].

1881 - Mikulicz [13](Fig - 24) and Leiter, adopted Max Nitze's principle of a rigid optical system and succeeded in constructing the first useful clinical gastroscope. Mikulicz also carried out numerous examinations on patients and obtained diagnostic results in Billroth's surgical clinic in Vienna. He was the first to use a miniature light bulb at the end of his gastroscope, which could be angled up to 30° at the third distal, thus anticipating the creation of the first semi-flexible gastroscope by more than 50 years. He described many modifications of surgical operations and he constructed the esophagoscope, scoliozymeter, and many other useful surgical devices. In 1881, he began research on constructing a device for endoscopy of the esophagus and stomach.In 1881, after the construction of the gastroscope with the help of Josef Leiter (1830-1892), a medical devices manufacturer; he became the first person in the world to diagnose cancer of the lower esophagus by endoscopy. Observations that he made concerning the endoscopic examination of patients with stomach cancer were published in 1883 in the *Przeglad Lekarski.* This work contains the world's first endoscopic description of gastric cancer.

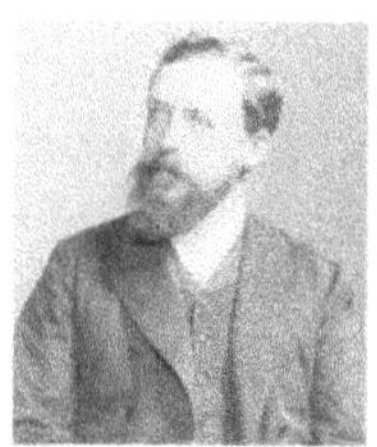

Fig – 24 Johann Anton von Mikulicz-Radecki (1850-1905) inventor of gastroscopy.

Howard Kelly (Fig - 25) described the first sigmoidoscopy in **1895**. The technique of examination utilized an electric light placed close to the patient s sacrum, and the light reflected off the examiner s head mirror.Further progress achieved by German surgeons was accomplished by Heinz Kalk (1895 - 1973) who, in 1929, introduced a new system of lenses for lateral vision at 45°. In 1935 he also published in the most important German medical journal, the 'Deutscher Medizinischer Wochenschrift', issue 46, his "dual trocar technique" of initiating and executing endoabdominal procedures. From 1929 to 1959 he published 21 works on laparoscopy. His monograph of 1951 reports his experience with over 2000 patients. The results were exceptional [14].In 1933 Fevers [15]. Used Kalk's technique while performing the first surgery on adhesiolysis with haemostasis through cauterization and in a few biopsies: this could be considered the first "modern" surgery using Laparoscopic Surgery. Fevers realised the risks of using oxygen to induce pneumoperitoneum and recommended the use of carbon dioxide [16]as an alternative. In 1937 a diagnosis of an ectopic pregnancy treated with laparoscopy was reported for the first time by the American Hope: it was the first use of Laparoscopic Surgery in emergency [17].

In a publication the following year Jano Veress, a Hungarian surgeon, reported that he had devised a needle to induce pneumoperitoneum, to drain the ascites and to drain air and liquid from the pleural cavities [18]. Veress' needle which is still used today has undergone few modifications in respect to the original.

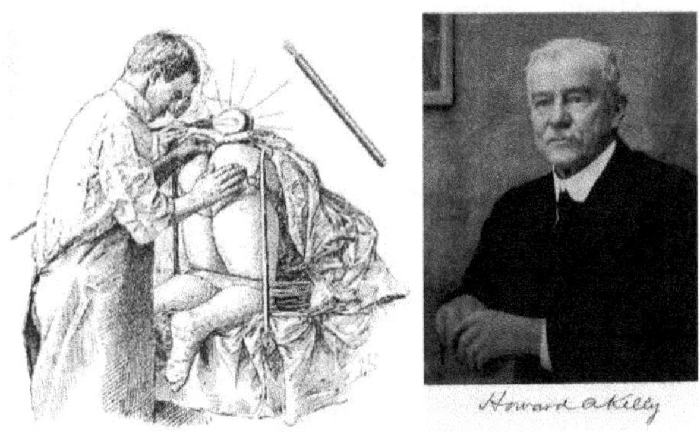

Fig - 25 Howard Atwood Kelly describing the technique of examination utilized an electric light placed close to the patient s sacrum, and the light reflected off the examiner's head mirror.

Grzegorz Litynski, a historian[19] at the Johann Wolfgang Goethe University in Frankfurt, profiled the key contributors in the history of laparoscopic surgery in a series of articles that appeared in the late **1990**s. Several important figures were in France and Germany during years surrounding World War II[20], a noteworthy commentary on the dedication of clinician scientists to their work in the midst of unimaginable political upheaval and social disruption. Many of

Litynski's references came from the European literature in the authors' native languages, so his articles are an important summary for English-only readers.

In **1887** using von Mikulicz's instrument, Gustav Killian performed the first bronchoscopies, increasing the illumination by using a small head mirror.

In **1901** George Kelling, (Fig - 26) of Dresden coined the term "colposcope" to describe the technique that using Nitze's cystoscope, insufflating it with oxygen filtered through sterile cotton wool, and coined the term "celioscopy" to examine the abdominal cavity and viewed the viscera of dogs. On September 23, 1901, he examined the peritoneal cavity of a dog. He was the first to examine the abdomen with an endoscope[21].

He found that insufflation of the abdomen with air, a procedure that he had tried in an unsuccessful attempt at controlling gastrointestinal haemorrhage, was a good way to create working space within the abdominal cavity. He reported these results at the German Biologic and Medical Society Meeting in Hamburg..Kelling also used filtered air to create a pneumoperitoneum, with the goal of stopping intra-abdominal bleeding (ectopic pregnancy, bleeding ulcers, and pancreatitis) but these studies did not find any response or supporters. Kelling noted that the abdominal cavity could store more than 2.5 liters of blood. The only method to establish a diagnosis and provide treatment at that time was linked to laparotomy. However, as Kelling observed, opening the abdomen could worsen the patient's condition.

To halt blood seepage into the abdomen, Kelling proposed a high-pressure insufflation of the abdominal cavity, a technique he called the "Lufttamponade" or "air tamponade"(Fig – 27) Working together with the Czech surgeon Vitezslav Chlumsky (Fig - 28) (1867-1943) in Breslau, Kelling expanded his insufflation technique. The purpose of his "coelioskope" was to view the effect of pneumoperitoneum acting as an air-tamponade and not as an endoscopic method itself. In the same year, Kelling presented the case to the Medical-Biological Society of Hamburg. He published it the following year. Kelling also used this technique to examine the abdomens of several patients, but he did not publish this experience immediately, limiting himself to describing it in letters to colleagues.

The only documentation of his experience was "a memorable lecture" before the Society of German Natural Scientists and Physicians in 1901 that predicted modern laparoscopy. He said, Endoscopic methods for the intestinal tract may find more use than it has been the case until now, as they are actually qualified to substitute the laparotomy in many cases.". He performed 45 such procedures to diagnose various lesions and tumours. Tragically, he died at age 79 in the Allied bombing of Dresden in 1945.

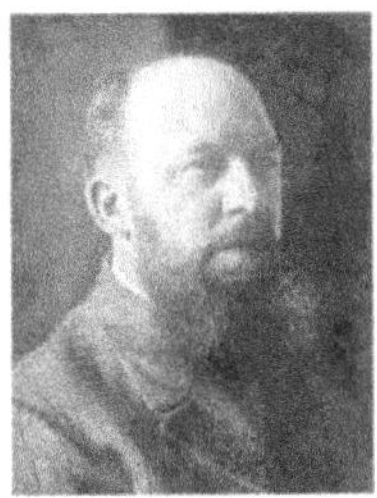

Fig – 26 George Kelling (1866-1945)

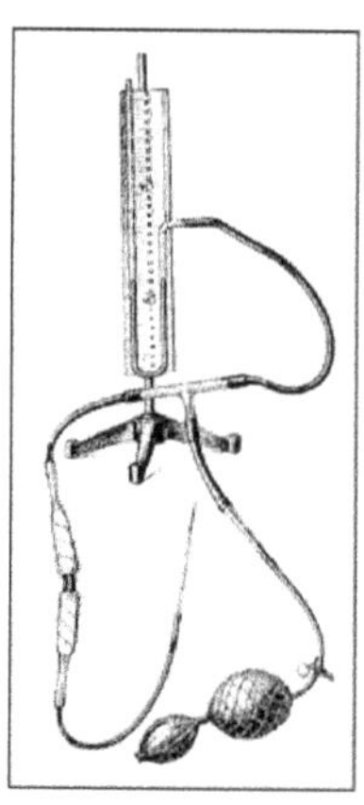

Fig 27 - An apparatus for Lufttamponade

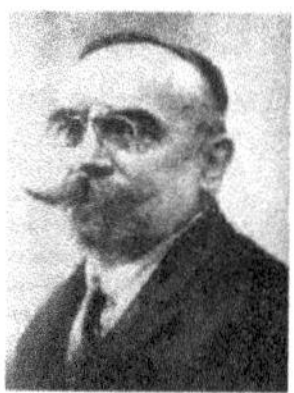

Fig - 28 Vitezslav Chlumsky , Czech surgeon and orthopedist , founder of the Czechoslovak Orthopedic Societ (1867-1943)

In the same year, **1901**, Dimitri Oskarovic von Ott (Fig – 29) from St. Petersburg examined the abdominal cavity of a pregnant woman using an illuminated head mirror. This was already not a celioscopy but a minilaparotomy . Dimitri Oscarovic Ott[22] (1855-1929) can be justified in calling himself one of the true pioneers of laparoscopy and especially of natural orifices transluminal endoscopic surgery (NOTES). As early as 1901 he performed abdominal examinations via a transvaginal access and called this procedure ventroscopy. The publication of his first results and a description of the method and equipment were released in 1902.

He was one of the pioneers of present day laparoscopy in addition to Georg Kelling (1866-1945) and Hans Christian Jacobaeus (1879-1937). He is regarded as the father of the Russian school of obstetrics and gynecology as well as founder of endoscopic surgery and laparoscopy in Russia.

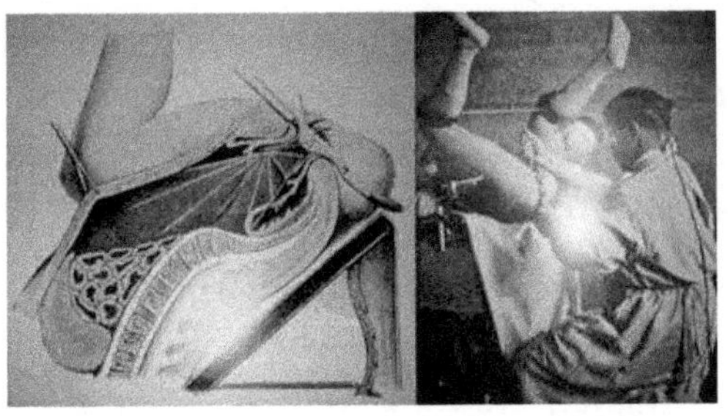

Fig – 29 Dimitri Oskarovic von Ott

In 1911 H.C. Jacobaeus (1879- 1937) (Fig – 30)from Stockholm, Sweden used for the first time the term "laparothorakoskopie" by using this procedure on the thorax and abdomen. He was an academic physician in Sweden who later became head of the department of internal medicine at the Karolinska Institute in 1916 and chair of its Nobel Prize committee, knew the necessity of publication to establish priority [23].

He also suggested employing a similar technique to examine body cavities endoscopically. He also did pioneer work involving abdominal endoscopy, which he called laparoscopy .He coined the term laparoscopy, deriving it from Greek. He called it initially as the"cystoscopy" of the serious cavities. He understood the possibilities, as well as the limitations of the procedure, and was an advocate of endoscopic training for medical personnel.

He also stressed the need for specialized instruments for optimum performance during laparoscopic examinations.

The first celioscopy performed on a human was carried out by him in 1901 using Nitze's cystoscope and without pneumoperitoneum[24].Despite the work of Cruise and Kelling, Jacobaeus has been called "the inventor of human laparoscopy and thoracoscopy." He performed diagnostic laparoscopy on 17 patients with ascites, an experience which he published in 1910.

He also examined two patients without ascites, a more difficult technical challenge where injury to the viscera was much higher. He took Kelling's idea of insufflation of air into the peritoneal cavity to create the distance to inspect intraabdominal structures, and used a trocar with a trap door that kept the air from escaping during the examination. He followed two years later with a second report of 97 patients, including 8 patients without ascites. In 1911 he performed 115 laparoscopies on 69 patients with only one serious complication (bleeding) which required a laparotomy.

In **1912** Jacobaeus began work with Ludolph Brauer at the Hamburg-Eppendorf Hospital in Germany and an advocate of therapeutic pneumothorax in the treatment of tuberculosis. In 1910, he published an article titled Über die Möglichkeit die Zystoskopie bei Untersuchung seröser Höhlungen anzuwenden (The Possibilities for Performing Cystoscopy in Examinations of Serous Cavities) in the journal Münchner

Medizinischen Wochenschrift[25]. They used thoracoscopy to free the lung from adhesions that prevented complete atelectasis.He largely abandoned laparoscopy, likely because the thoracoscopy allowed a therapeutic intervention, whereas the conditions where he used laparoscopy were mostly incurable, such as liver disease and malignancy.

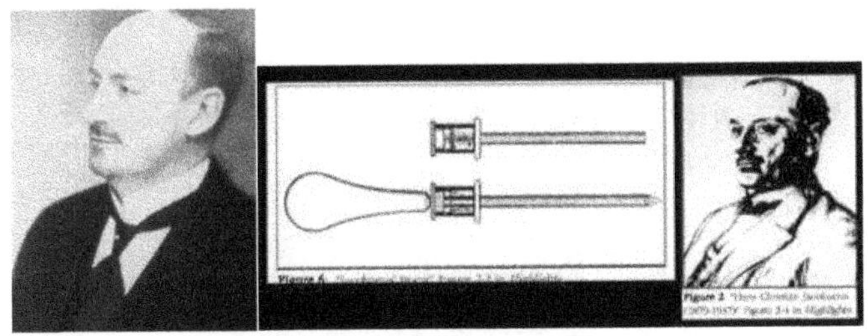

Fig – 30 Hans Christian Jacobaeus , professor at the Karolinska Institutet in Stockholm. From 1925 – 1937.

In **1911**, one year after Jacobaeus's report, Bertram Bernheim (Fig – 31) of Baltimore The instrument he called organoscopy [26]was a proctoscope of a half inch diameter and ordinary light for illumination. He used a 12mm proctoscope, inserted in the epigastrium in order to study a patient with a pancreatic tumor and appendicitis, and published the first American article on laparoscopy. He reported the use of a sigmoidoscope in United States of America to inspect the interior of the abdomen.

After working the procedure out on dogs at the Hunterian Laboratory at Johns Hopkins, he tried it on two human patients, one on a jaundiced patient with a distended gall bladder from a carcinoma at the head of the pancreas; the other, a patient suspected of a chronic gastric ulcer who had chronic appendicitis. With such modest results, Bernheim's interests turned to other areas. In addition to this, acting on the theory that nothing definite has been found in a given case, we have drawn a part the stomach out through the wound, made an incision in its anterior wall[27], and inserted the cystoscope directly into its cavity. A stomach tube passed in through the mouth acts as a guide in this procedure and aids in a careful inspection of the whole gastric mucosa. On withdrawing the cystoscope, the wound in the stomach is closed in the usual way.

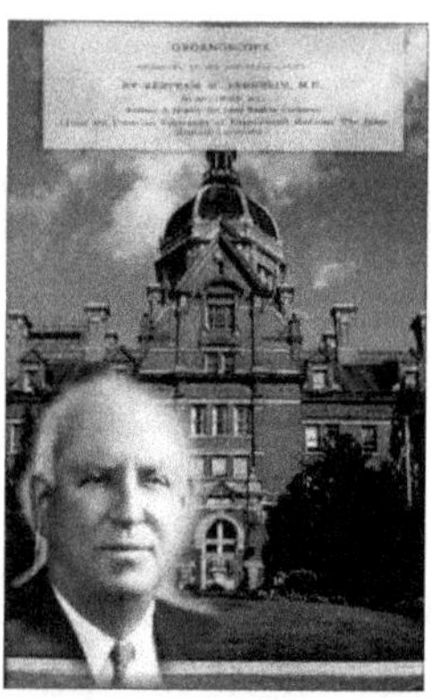

Fig – 31 Bertram M. Bernheim, Johns Hopkins University. School of Medicine. Baltimore, Maryland. The United States (1955).

New Yorkers Arthur Stein, a gynecologist, and William Stewart, a radiologist, introduced the modality in America in **1919**. They used an anaesthesia bag to inflate the free abdominal cavity in **1921**, Walter Alvarez, an internist in San Francisco, reported the use of carbon dioxide for the procedure.

The peritoneal cavity absorbed carbon dioxide within a few minutes, a distinct advantage over oxygen or air, which sometimes remained in the abdomen over days with prolonged discomfort.

In 1920 the American William R. Orndorff added the typical pyramidal points to this instrument, in order to facilitate the insertion [28].

Benjamin Orndoff, in1920s from Chicago (Fig - 32) the founding chair of the department of radiology at the Stritch College of Medicine at the Loyola University in Chicago, familiar with the diagnostic pneumoperitoneum, tried his hand at laparoscopy and reported his experience in **1921**. What induced him, as a radiologist, to probe the secrets of the unopened abdomen with a technique he called "peritoneoscopy" is not clear. First, he began by using a pharyngoscope or a cystoscope with a lamp and lens system in animals to learn the method. Later, he used a modification of the more sophisticated instrument devised by Hans Christian Jacobeus in Sweden. He induced a pneumoperitoneum through an intraspinal needle with oxygen under local anesthesia. His penchant for radiology then took over [29]. He fluoroscoped the abdomen to determine the relative distention of the peritoneal cavity and to locate pathological organs, which it would be desirable to avoid when the peritoneoscope is inserted. He then inserted his trocar and cannula, threading his peritoneoscope through the cannula to make his observations.

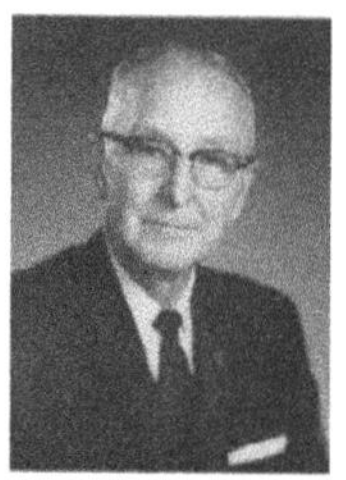

Fig – 32 Benjamin Harry Orndoff, M.D.1881–1971

Reports of similar experiences arrived from Denmark, Finland, France, Italy, Hungary, and Brazil, confirming the spread of the technique. In **1935** he also published in the most important German medical journal, the 'Deutscher Medizinischer Wochenschrift', issue 46, his "dual trocar technique" of initiating and executing endo abdominal procedures. From **1929 to 1959** he published 21 works on laparoscopy. His monograph of 1951 reports his experience with over 2000 patients.

He was just the exemplary pioneer, paid particular attention to defining and articulating the precise contraindications for laparoscopy, definitions which had never really been categorized thoroughly at this time. He recognized laparoscopy potential but also recognized the need for more training and information on the subject.

Orndoff was also was the one who coined the term peritoneoscopy. In addition to his incredible clinical success, Orndoff is also well known for his (1920) report on 42 peritoneoscopies, which was one of the first large published series of its kind. He also made several technical innovations, including a sharp pyramidal trocar point that allowed for greater ease for the initial trocar puncturing.

He changed from using regular atmospheric air to the purer (but less stable) element of oxygen. He had accumulated 42 clinical cases, on the basis of which he published in his seminal article, “The Peritoneoscope in the Diagnosis of Diseases of the Abdomen.”4 He described his observations on patients with localized and generalized peritonitis, hemoperitoneum, ascites, ectopic pregnancy, salpingitis, ovarian tumors, and intra-abdominal neoplasms of various kinds, including carcinomas of the stomach, pancreas, and hematologic malignancies.

In the annals of the history of laparoscopy, he is all but ignored. Not until the mid-1930s was laparoscopy resurrected by Dr John C. Ruddock of Los Angeles. Even thereafter, it languished as a rarely used diagnostic tool until the mid-1970s, when advances in optics and instrumentation dramatically increased its usage in the United States.

Many technical developments which increased safety and efficacy were introduced during this formative stage that helped laparoscopy to become a more accepted procedure. In **1912**, Severine Nordentoft, a gynecologist from Copenhagen, was the first to adopt the position of Trendelenburg for laparoscopy.

In 1918 O. Goetze, (Fig – 33) developed an automatic pneumoperitoneum needle characterized for its safe introduction to the peritoneal cavity. In 1921, two German surgeons further improved laparoscopy: R. Korbsch described and adopted the needle to induce pneumoperitoneum and Otto Goetze invented the apparatus for insufflation [30'31]

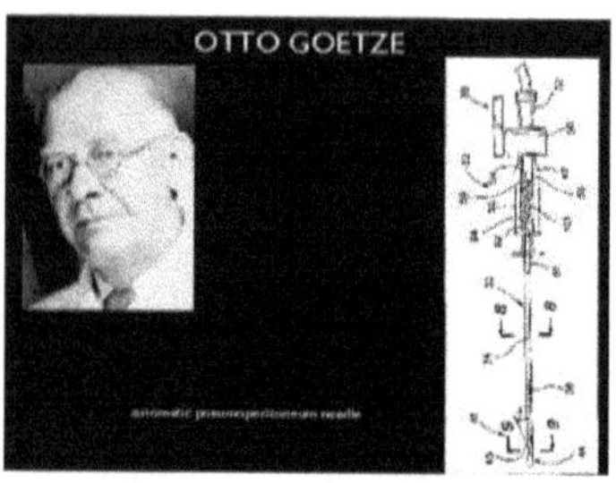

Fig – 33 O. Goetze

Stewart and Stein have having introduced laparoscopy into the US in **1919.** In **1920** the American William R. Orndorff added the typical pyramidal points to this instrument, in order to facilitate the insertion. In **1920**, Zollikofer of Switzerland discovered the benefit of CO2 gas to use for insufflation, rather than filtered atmospheric air or nitrogen. The first needle for the introduction of a pneumoperitoneum was done by Korbsch in **1921**. The later invention of the insufflator was done by Goetze also in **1921**.

A new optics system in **1923** was invented by Unverricht who was instrumental in designing a lens system with a widened viewing angle through the laparoscope.. Zollikofer's done the introduction of CO2 as a means for insufflations [32] in **1924**.

Basil Hirschowitz (Fig – 34) (**1925**) further developed the fiberoptic system, and in February **1957** performed the first fiberoptic gastroscopy on a patient a few days after he had passed the gastroscope into his own stomach.

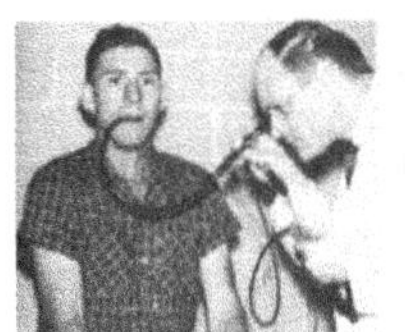 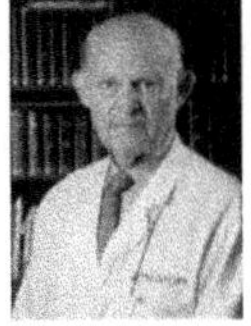

Fig – 34 Basil Hirschowitz, Bethal, South Africa (1925 –2013)

This instrument diminished patient discomfort by enhancing flexibility and by reducing bulk. Notable endoscope refinements of the late 1960s and early 1970s included re-positioning of lenses for wider field of vision, addition of channels for biopsy forceps, suction, air, or water, and four-way controlled tip deflection. The expanding diagnostic capabilities of endoscopy were soon complemented by new therapeutic applications, including colon polypectomy with a wire loop snare (1971), cannulation of the pancreatic duct (1972), removal of biliary stone (1975), and placement of feeding tubes by gastrostomy (1979). The range of technical developments in gastrointestinal endoscopy was so extensive across a broad front that John F. Morrissey was prompted to claim that "I think we are approaching a plateau in instrument development."

Laparoscopy development during World war (Europe)

In **1929 Heinz Kalk,** (Fig – 35) a German gastroenterologist is considered the founder of the German School of Laparoscopy. Kalk developed a forward-looking oblique 135-degree lens system and a dual-trocar approach. He studied surgery at the Charité

Hospital in Berlin after serving in World War I on the Western Front. Because the liver and spleen lay beyond the diagnostic capabilities of gastroscopy and radiology, he became interested in diagnostic laparoscopy. He in 1929 introduced a new system of lenses for lateral vision at 45°.He used laparoscopy as a diagnostic method for liver and gallbladder disease. He developed a dual-trocar technique and a wide-angle scope to obtain biopsies. In 1939 he publishes his experience of 2000 liver biopsies performed using local anaesthesia without mortality. He advocated the use of a separate puncture site for pneumoperitoneum. In **1935** he also published in the most important German medical journal, the 'Deutscher Medizinischer Wochenschrift', issue 46, his "dual-trocar technique" of initiating and executing endo abdominal procedures.

From **1929 to 1959** he published 21 works on laparoscopy. His monograph of 1951 reports his experience with over 2000 patients. The results were exceptional. In 1928 he obtained a special endoscope with a 135-degree field of view. He designed a trocar that had a spring device that retracted its sharp point after entry, a principle much like the Veres needle. By 1942 he had performed 750 procedures, including biopsies of the spleen (which he first did in 1934), and liver (in 1935, reporting 123 biopsies in 1943).

He was in the medical services of the Luftwaffe in World War II(Fig – 32), where he put his device to use in performing diagnostic laparoscopies on soldiers suffering from epidemic hepatitis. With the Nazi attack on the Soviet Union in 1941, German troops began to contract hepatitis in large numbers. The spread of epidemic hepatitis among German soldiers caused Kalk to take a serious look at liver biopsy. The high fatality rate of blind liver biopsy, then standard practice, convinced Kalk to turn to laparoscopic biopsy. In 1942 and 1943, Kalk perfected the technique of laparoscopic liver biopsy and introduced the procedure in military hospitals throughout German-occupied Europe[33].

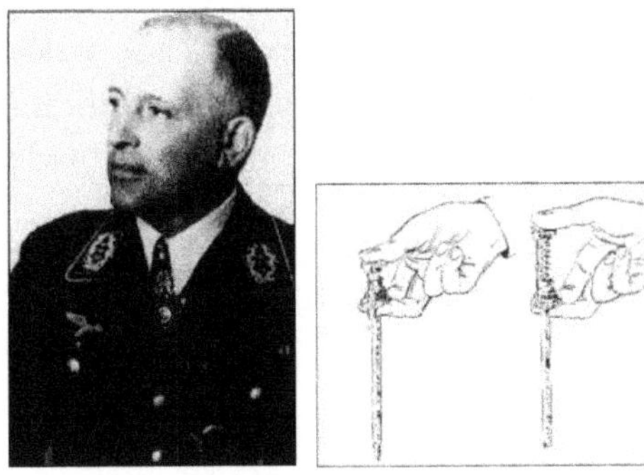

Fig – 35 Heinz Kalk (1895 – 1973 1939 - Kalk's trocar was working Luftwaffe, the German air force.

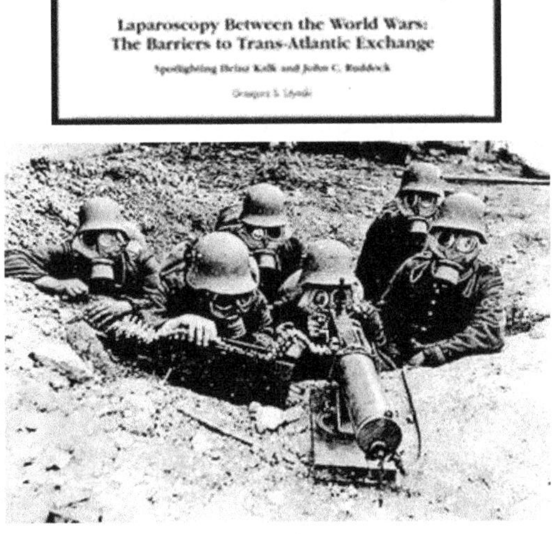

Fig - 36 World War II

The first textbook on laparoscopy and thoracoscopy was published In 1927 by Korbsch [34].

In **1933** Fevers used Kalk's technique while performing the first surgery on adhesiolysis with haemostasis through cauterization and in a few biopsies: this could be considered the first "modern" surgery using Laparoscopic Surgery. Fevers realised the risks of using oxygen to induce pneumoperitoneum and recommended the use of carbon dioxide as an alternative.

Laparoscopy development during World war (U.S.A)

On the American side, **John Ruddock** (Fig - 37) in Los Angeles had done more than 2,500 laparoscopic surgeries and taken 1,000 biopsies between wars in the **1930s and 1940s**. In 1934, he described laparoscopic as a good diagnostic method, many times, superior to laparotomy. His instrument consisted of a built-in forceps with electrocoagulatio capacity. He used a McCarthy cystoscope that he had modified to include a redesigned trocar with biopsy instruments. He also introduced local anesthesia to facilitate the procedure. In 1937, he reported on his initial experiences with 500 patients (background), and by the time he retired, he had performed more than 2500 laparoscopies with much success and low morbidity. In 1949 he reported a diagnostic accuracy of nearly 94 percent. Ruddock, like Kalk, had served in the armed forces in both wars. Contemporaries and pioneers in the same field, they faced impossible barriers of language, geography, politics, and ultimately armed conflict. Kalk and Ruddock's enthusiasm for the procedure was not generally held, especially among surgeons. It made little sense to perform laparoscopy under general anesthesia simply for diagnosis, when one could do a definitive operation through a standard incision. A survey of internists and surgeons taken in 1966 documented that less than 10 percent had done a diagnostic laparoscopic procedure, and fewer than one percent had done more than . "After a brief stir," wrote Litynski, "most surgeons abandoned peritoneoscopy because of its limited therapeutic applications." Ruddock presented his peritoneoscope for the first time in 1934. The term "peritoneoscopy" was initially proposed by Orndoff of Chicago in 1920.[35]

Ruddock's instrument consisted of a fluid evacuator equipped with an air-tight lock, a pneumoperitoneum needle, sheath and bistoury-tipped obturator which acted as a trocar, "Telescope" (14-inch, preoblique optic), and biopsy forceps.[36]Robert Hope, who assisted Ruddock for three years, examined the use of peritoneoscopy for diagnosing extra-uterine pregnancy.[37]Edward Benedict of Boston described the aspiration of an ovarian cyst under peritoneoscopic view.[38]William Lee of Philadelphia performed cholecystography under peritoneoscopic examination.[39]Robinson and Fiske of Santa Barbara, California, presented a retractor for displacing viscera during peritoneoscopic examination.[40] "Peritoneoscopy has received much more attention during the past year than ever before," summarized Beling in 1941.[41]After the first World War, and about the same time, John C. Ruddock left the United States Navy to enter private practice in Los Angeles. However he concentrated on cardiology in the 1920s. He was an active member of the American College of Cardiology and, in 1931, became president of the California Heart Association.[42]

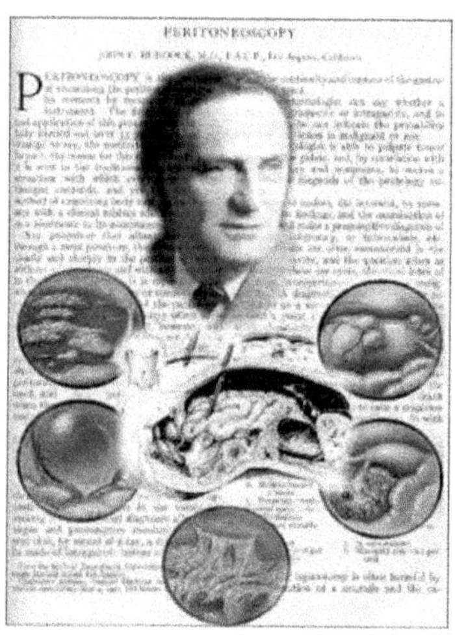

(Fig – 37) John Ruddock (1891-1964)

Kalk and Ruddock overcame the technological limitations of the 1920s to create usable instruments with a graded optical system. They were also able to determine clear indications and contraindications for laparoscopy. Although very similar in appearance, the development of laparoscopic instruments and investigatory methods took different paths in Europe and the United States. In **1937** Hope R (USA) Published the diagnosis of an ectopic pregnancy treated with laparoscopy was reported for the first time: it was the first use of Laparoscopic Surgery in an emergency

Referrences

1. Lau WY, Leow CK, Li AK. History of endoscopic and laparoscopic surgery. *World J Surg.* 1997;21:444–453.

2. David TE. Innovation in surgery. *J Thorac Cardiovasc Surg.* 2000;119(suppl):38–41.

3. Darwin C. *On the Origin of Species by Means of Natural Selection, or the Preservation of Favoured Races in the Struggle for Life.* London: John Murray, 1859.

4. Development of the Modern Cystoscope: An Illustrated History,Rainer Engel, MD,October 24, 2007

5. Johnson SK, Naidu RK, Ostopowicz RC, et al. Adolf Kussmaul: distinguished clinician and medical pioneer. *Clin Med Res* 2009; 7: 107–112.

6. Killian H (1901) Dtsch. Z. Chir. 58,499 .

7. Proc R Soc Med. 1969 Aug; 62(8): 781–786.,Origins of Oesophagology.H. D. Kelly

8. Nitze M. Eine neue Beobachtungs- und Untersuchungsmethode für Harnröhre, Harnblase und Rektum. Wien. Med Wschr 1879;29:649-652.

9. Matthias Reuter, Hans J. Reuter, Rainer Engel: *History of Endoscopy*, pp 159-275.

10. Matthias Reuter, Hans J. Reuter, Rainer Engel: *History of Endoscopy*, pp 159-275.

11. Nezhat, Dr. Camran, and Barbara Page. "THE LARYNX ILLUMINATED." 'History of Endoscopy' Ed. Dr. Paul Alan Wetter. Society of Laproendoscopic Surgeons, 1 Jan. 2005. Web. 16 Mar. 2015.

12. Surg Endosc 2007: 21; 838-853 Springer Verlag)

13. Mikulicz J.,Resekcja odźwiernika z powodu raka. Wyleczenie. Uwagi nad pewnym objawem raka żołądkowego, za pomocą gastroskopu spostrzegać się dającym.Przegląd Lekarski. 1883; 22: 157-158

14. Kalk H, Bruhl W. Leitfaden der Laparoskopie und Gastroskopie. Thieme Stuttgard. 1951..

15. Gotz F, Pier A, Schippers E, Schumpelick V. The history of laparoscopy. In: Gotz F, Pier A, Schippers E, Schumpelick V, editors. Color Atlas of Laparoscopic Surgery. New York 1993:3-

16. Fervers, C., Die Laparoskopie mit dem Cystoskop. Ein Beitrag zur Vereinfachung der Technik und zur endoskopischen Strangdurchtrennung in der Bauchhöhle. Med Klin 1933; 29:1042-1045

17. Hope R. The differential diagnosis of ectopic pregnancy by peritoneoscopy. Surg Gynecol Obst 1937;64:229-232.

18. Veress J. Neues Instrument zur Ausführung von Brust-oder Bauchpunktionen und Pneumothoraxbehandlung. Deut Med Wschr 1938;64: 1480–1483.

19. Laparoscopy - The Early Attempts: Spotlighting Georg Kelling and Hans Christian Jacobaeus,Grzegorz S. Litynski

20. JSLS.(Journal of the society of laparoscopic & Robotic surgeons) 1997 Jan-Mar; 1(1): 83–85.

21. Kelling G. Mittelung zur Benutzung des Oesophagoscops. *Allgemeine Medicinsche Central-Zeitung*. 1896; 65: 73

22. Geschichte der Urologie,Published: 30 June 2013,Dimitrij Oscarovic Ott (1855–1929) „Die Ventroskopie"- Springer.

23. Journal of Endourology Hans Christian Jacobaeus: Inventor of Human Laparoscopy and Thoracoscopy

24. Jacobaeus HC. Ueber die Möglichkeit die Zystoskopie bei Untersuchungen seröser Höhlungen anzuwenden. Munch Med Wochenschr. 1910;**57**:2090–2019.

25. JSLS. 1997 Jan-Mar; 1(1): 83–85. Laparoscopy - The Early Attempts: Spotlighting Georg Kelling and Hans Christian Jacobaeus,Grzegorz S. Litynski.

26. ORGANOSCOPY. CYSTOSCOPY OF THE ABDOMINAL CAVITY. BY BERTRAM M. BERNHEIM, M.D., OF

BALTIMORE, MD., Assistant in Surgery, The Johns Hopkins University. (From the Hunterian Laboratory of Experimental Medicine, The Johns Hopkins University.) Ann Surg. 1911 Jun; 53(6): 764–767.

27. Expanding the role of the educator into organizational development.*Carpenter D, Davis R,Nurs Staff Dev Insid. 1995 Mar-Apr; 4(2):3.*
28. Orndorff BH. The peritoneoscope in diagnosis of diseases of the abdomen. J Radiol 1920;1:307–310.
29. An Unlikely Pioneer in Laparoscopy: Benjamin Henry Orndoff, MD Leon Morgenstern, MD, FACS.Surgical Innovation Volume 15 Number 1 March 2008 5-6 © 2008 Sage Publications
30. Korbsch R. Die Laparoskopie nach Jacobaeus. Berl Klin Wschr 1921;58:696-700.
31. Goetz O. Ein neues Verfahren zur Gasfüllung für das Pneumoperitoneum. Münch Med Wschr 1921;51:233-236.
32. Zollikofer R. Zur Laparoskopie. Schw Med Wochenschr. 1924;**54**:264.
33. Wildhirt E. Heinrich-Otto Kalk 1895-1973. Lebensbild eines gastroeneterologen und hepatologen. *Falk Foundation*, 1995
34. The first textbook on laparoscopy and thoracoscopy was published In 1927 by Korbsch.
35. Orndoff BH. The peritoneoscope in diagnosis of disease of the abdomen. *J Rad.* 1920;l:307–325
36. Ruddock JC. Peritoneoscopy. *West J Surg.* 1934;42:392–405
37. Hope RB. The differential diagnosis of ectopic gestation by peritoneoscopy. *Surg Gyne Obstet.* 1937;64:229–234
38. Benedict EB. Peritoneoscopy. *New Engl J Med.* 1938;218:713–719
39. Lee WY. Evaluation of peritoneoscopy in intra-abdominal diagnosis. *Rev Gastroenterol* 1942;9:133–141

40. Robinson S, Fiske LG. An instrument for retraction of viscera during peritoneoscopy. *West J Surg Obstet Gynecol.* 1941:284-288

41. Beling CA. Selection of cases for peritoneoscopy. *Arch Surg.* 1941;41:872-889

42. The National Cyclopedia of American Biography. *Current Series*, Vol G Ann Arbor: Xerox, 1967

5.World War II to 1960 AD

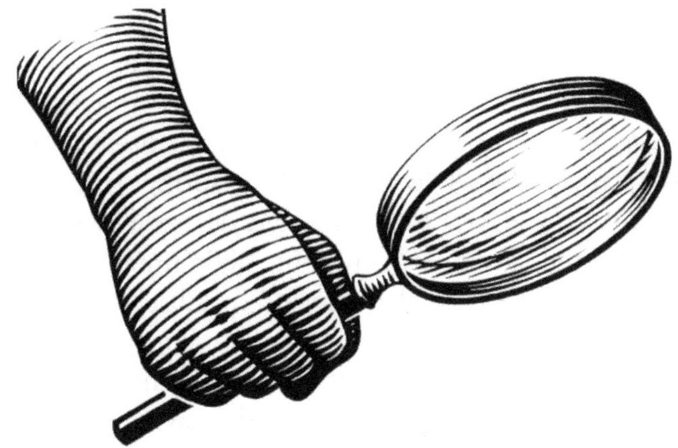

In1938 **Janos Veress**[1] (Fig -38), of a Hungarian internist, developed the spring-loaded needle.He described his eponymic needle in a 1936 report in the Hungarian literature in a description of inducing pneumothorax for tuberculosis. To protect the organs from injury, he placed a spring loaded blunt obturator within a needle. The wall of the chest or abdomen pushed the blunt tipped obturator backward, exposing the sharp edge of the needle and allowing the assembly to penetrate the layers of tissue. When the tip of the needle entered a body cavity, the sudden loss of tissue resistance allowed the obturator to spring forward beyond the end of the needle, where it could protect the underlying viscera from injury. Its main purpose was to perform therapeutic pneumothorax to treat patients suffering from tuberculosis. He used it to drain the ascites and to drain air and liquid from the pleural cavities. Its current modifications make the "Veress" needle a perfect tool to achieve pneumoperitoneum during laparoscopic surgery. Interestingly, Veress did not promote the use of his Veress needle for laparoscopy purposes. He used a veress needle for the induction of pneumothorax. It consists of an outer cannula with a beveled needle point for cutting through tissues. Inside the cannula of a verse, needle is an inner stylet, the stylet is loaded with a spring that spring forward in response to the sudden decrease in pressure encountered upon crossing the abdominal wall and entering the peritoneal cavity.Alfred Cuschieri, one of the leading figures of surgical laparoscopy, speculated that Kurt Semm was one of the first to use the Veres needle in his pioneering work on laparoscopic surgery.Veress' needle which is still used today, has undergone few modifications in respect to the original.

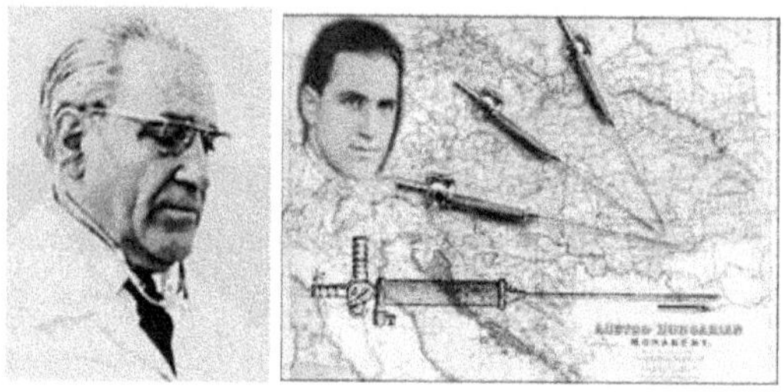

Fig – 38 Janos Veress, a Hungarian physician (1938)

In **1939, Richard Wesley Telinde** [2](Fig – 39) tried to perform an endoscopic procedure by a culdoscopic approach, in the lithotomy position. This method was rapidly abandoned because of the presence of small intestine.

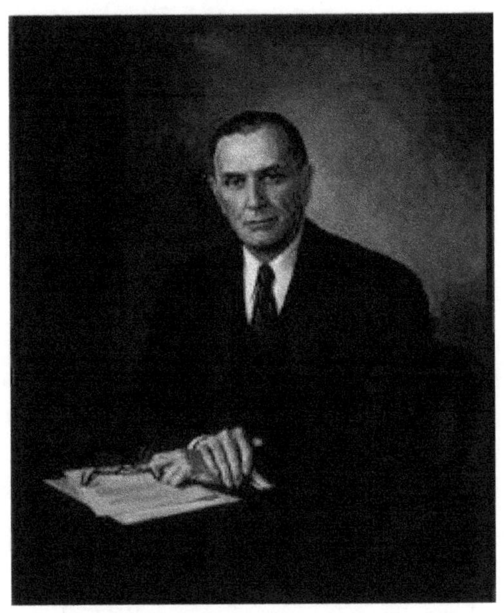

Fig – 39 Telinde Richard Wesley (1894 - 1989)

In **1944 Raoul Palmer**(Fig – 40), a gynecologist at the Hôpital Broca in Paris, and his wife Elizabeth started to perform laparoscopic procedures in 1943.He performed gynecological examinations using laparoscopy and placing the patients in the Trendelenburg position, so air could fill the pelvis. He also stressed the importance of continuous intra-abdominal pressure monitoring during a laparoscopic procedure.

He introduced the most popular method of the closed laparoscopic entry in **1947** Use of the Veress needle to induce CO2 pneumoperitoneum for laparoscopy Published on its safety in the first 250 patients.

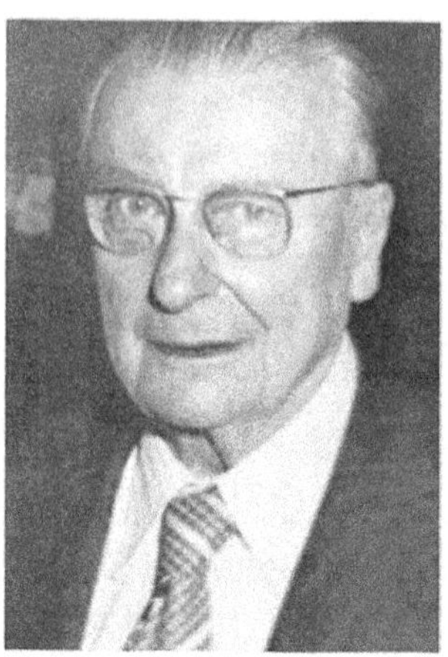

Fig – 40 Raoul Palmer (1905–1985), Paris.

As the war drew to a close everything became scarce, from household items to hospital supplies. Raoul recognized the importance of controlling the amount of pressure within the abdomen, so he added a manometer to his insufflator. He was unable to drive to nearby towns because of gasoline rationing, he rode his bicycle seek to obtain the carbonic acid necessary to generate carbon dioxide gas. Surgical gloves were in short supply, so the Palmers rinsed their hands repeatedly with an alcohol solution during their procedures.The Palmers first used cystoscopes outfitted with incandescent bulbs the size of a corn kernel. Attached to a 4.5 V flashlight battery outfitted with a rheostat, they often burned out during examinations. Despite the challenges of wartime, in **1947** Palmer reported an experience of 250 "coelioscopies gynecologiques"[3] that included descriptions of his instrumentation and examination techniques, "the most substantial published work on the application of laparoscopy in women's medicine at the time." The miniature light bulbs barely gave enough light to examine the pelvic organs, much less photography. In 1952 a Parisian optical firm used quartz rods to transfer light from a 150 V lamp outside the body. Despite its shortcomings - the lamp was "very hot," it needed a cooling system so noisy that it made normal conversation impossible, and the quartz rods were fragile and broke easily - it was the most effective means of illumination until fibre optic cold light systems became available in the 1960s. It was the proximal illumination, provided enough light for photography; the Palmers even made an 8 mm colour movie of a procedure in **1955**. Added to his expertise in infertility, laparoscopy made Raoul Palmer a leading international figure in gynecology.

The next decade and a half saw interruption of technological advances and a lack of any substantial development in endoscopy due to World War I (Fig - **41) and II** (Fig - 42)(1900 -1918) and (1939 - 1945)

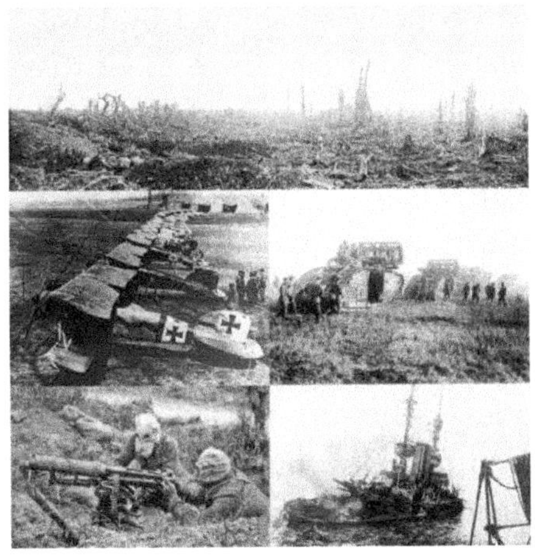

World war 1 Fig - 41)

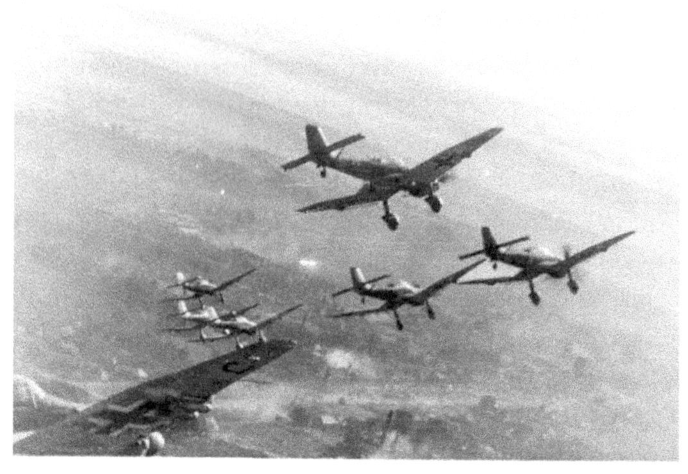

World war II (Fig - 42)

In **1953, Harold Hopkins and Narinder Singh Kapany** (Fig - 44)at Imperial College in London succeeded in making image-transmitting bundles with over 10,000 fibers, and subsequently achieved image transmission through a 75 cm long bundle which combined several thousand fibers.[4][5][6] The first practical fiber optic semi-flexible gastroscope was patented by Basil Hirschowitz, C. Wilbur Peters, and Lawrence E. Curtiss, researchers at the University of Michigan, in 1956. In the process of developing the gastroscope, Curtiss produced the first glass-clad fibers; previous optical fibers had relied on air or impractical oils and waxes as the low-index cladding material.[16]

Narinder Singh Kapany Often described as the 'father of fiber optics,' who introduced the term in a 1960 article in *Scientific American*[7], wrote the first book about the new field, and played a prominent role in advancing the field both as a researcher and as the founder of several optical technology companies.

Harold Hopkins (Fig - 43) applied fiberoptics to endoscopy, and invented a new rod-lens optical system in **1954**. This invention led to the era of modern endoscopy. The Hopkins glass rod-lens, developed by him in the late 1950s, produced images 80 times better than the Galilean optics that had been used in traditional cystoscopes. Fiber optics originated in the same decade with papers published back-to-back in Nature in 1954 by Hopkins and Narinder Karpany (Fig -44) at the University College in London and their rival, Abraham van Heel, at the University of Delft. Lawrence Curtiss at the University of Michigan made a key improvement by cladding each fiber with glass of a lower refractive index, which prevented the loss of light by assuring internal reflection along the length of the light-carrying fiber.

Fiber optics made two fundamental technological contributions to medicine: flexible endoscopy and proximal illumination. The former revolutionized the practice of gastroenterology; the latter provided the light needed for laparoscopic surgery. The principle was the same as the Palmer's arrangement with a high voltage light source outside the body, but now illuminated glass fibers placed on the rim of the endoscope brought light inside the body, and thus replaced the Palmers' unwieldy quartz rods.

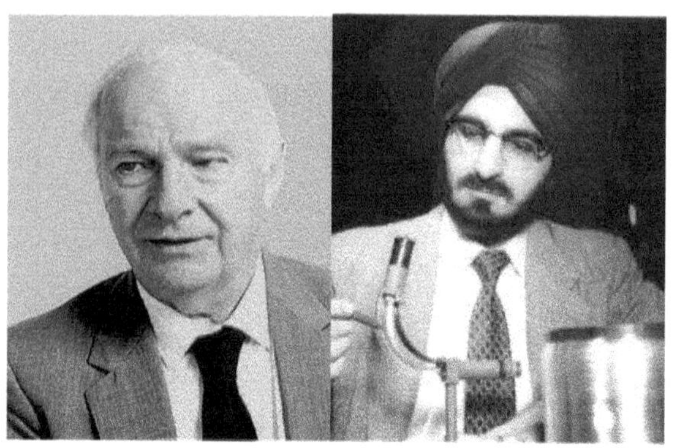

Fig – 43 Harold Hopkins (1918–1995) Fig – 44 Dr. Narinder Singh Kapany (1926-2020)

However, the real revolution is only very recent and dates back to the early 1950s, with the use of fiber optics that allowed the resolution of the main obstacles. A revolutionary development was the introduction of cold light fiberglass illumination, the product of the efforts of French scientist Max Fourestier and his colleagues in 1952 [8]. Since then, technical progress has continued to follow, especially with the advent of video-endoscopy. Visualization improved remarkably with the Hopkins lens and fibreoptic cold illumination; however, interest in these techniques waned for several decades.

Harold Horace Hopkins obtained a degree in physics and mathematics at Leicester University in 1939. After the war, in 1947, Hopkins became a research fellow at Imperial College, London, UK. Hopkins invented the rigid rod-lens system for scopes, which allows double light transmission, requires short and thin spacer tubes, and gives a larger and clearer aperture. He filed a patent for the rod-lens system in 1959. However, the English and American companies to whom he offered the system displayed little interest. The situation changed however in 1965 when Professor George Berci, who recognized the potential of this invention, introduced Hopkins to Karl Storz to manufacture the scopes[9].

By the 1970s Hopkins' quartz rod-lens had evolved into a "flexible fiber optic" made from thousands of glass fibers[10].Small one- or two-man inventors were now being supported in collaboration with expert teams from companies such as "Storz, Olympus, ACMI, and Philips"[11]. The work of Hopkins and his coworkers formed the basis for flexible fiber-optic endoscopes and modern rigid laparoscopes.

Modern endoscopy developed basically overnight toward the technology currently being used. It is easy to understand this immediate jump toward modernity due to "clear and color-true images, with a breathtaking 3- D like field of vision with a depth of field never before imagined" [11].In **1952** the same year three Frenchmen, N. Fourestier, A. Gladu and J. Vulmiere were the first to adopt this new system of illumination for laparoscopy (cold light laparoscopy) .

Refereences

1. Szabó, István; László, Ádám (2004). "Veres Needle: In Memoriam of the 100th Birthday Anniversary of Dr János Veres, the Inventor". American Journal of Obstetrics & Gynecology. **191** (1): 352–3.
2. Obstet Gynecol, 1959 Aug;14(2):257-66.,A visit with Dr. Richard Wesley Te Linde- S G BERKOW

3. Instrumentation and technique of gynecological laparoscopy.PALMER R - Gynecol Obstet (Paris). 1947; 46(4):420-31.

4. *Hecht, Jeff (2004). City of Light: The Story of Fiber Optics (revised ed.). Oxford University. pp. 55–70.*

5. Hopkins, H. H. & Kapany, N. S. (1954). "A flexible fibrescope, using static scanning". *Nature*. **173** (4392): 39–41.

6. Two Revolutionary Optical Technologies. Scientific Background on the Nobel Prize in Physics 2009. Nobelprize.org. 6 October 2009

7. "Asian American Pacific Islander Heritage Month: The Father of Fiber Optics". Transportation History. 3 May 2017. Archived from the original on 12 June 2020. Retrieved 12 June 2020

8. Fourestier, M., Gladu, A., and Vulmière, J. 1952. Perfectionnements à l'endoscopie médicale. Réalisation bronchoscopique. *La Presse Médicale* 60:1292–1294.).

9. (Courtesy of William P. Didusch Center for Urologic History, American Urological Association, MD, USA)

10. Powers, Clarice J. "A Brief History of Endoscopy." Seminars in Perioperative Nursing 2.3 (1993): 129-32.

11. Nezhat, Dr. Camran, and Barbara Page. "1970'S." 'History of Endoscopy' Ed. Dr. Paul Alan Wetter. Society of Laproendoscopic Surgeons, 1 Jan. 2005. Web. 16 Mar. 2015

6. 1960 AD to Recent times

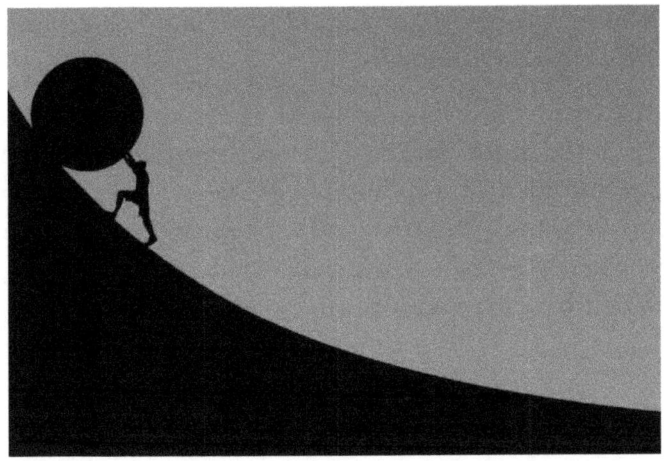

In1960 **Kurt Karl Stephan Semm**[1] (1927-2003) (Fig -45),a German who invented the automatic insufflator. His experience with this new device was published in **1966**. Although not recognized in his own land, on the other side of the Atlantic, both American physicians and instrument makers valued the Semm for the automatic insufflator which monitored abdominal pressure, and its simple application, clinical value, and safety. In **1966**, he introduced automatic insufflator. This allowed for safer laparoscopy and avoids bowel perforations and retroperitoneal vascular injuries. Semm developed thermocoagulation, irrigation devices. He adapted numerous surgical procedures to laparoscopic techniques, including tubal sterilization, salpingostomy, oophorectomy, salpingolysis, and tumor reduction therapy. Beyond the realm of gynecologic surgery, Semm popularized laparoscopic procedures, such as omental adhesiolysis, bowel suturing, tumor biopsy, and staging, and, notably, incidental appendectomy in **1983** and from 1970 to 1991 Semm performed more than 20.000 pelvi scopes, replacing 70% of the laparotomies.

Over all in 1970s, as the Head of Gynecology in Kiel, introduced an; 1- Automatic insufflation device capable of monitoring intra-abdominal pressures, 2- Endoscopic loop sutures, 3-Extra- and intracorporeal suturing techniques. 4-Created the pelvi- trainer. He performed the first laparoscopic appendectomy [2]in 1982.

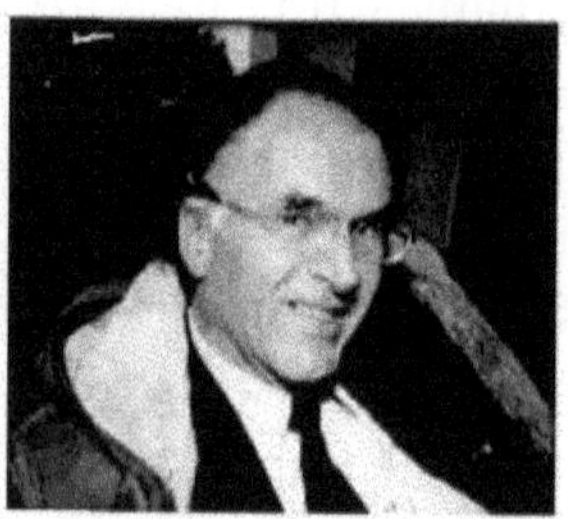

Kurt Karl Stephan Semm (1927–2003)

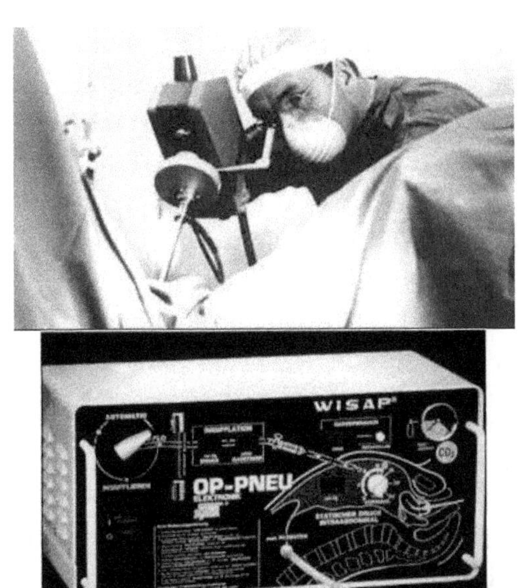

Fig -45 .Kurt Semm (1927–2003) Semm performing video laparoscopy.

He developed the hook scissors, the endoloop applicator, the pre-tied loop (Roeder loop), the high volume irrigation/aspiration apparatus, the laparoscopic thermocoagulation, the instrument for macro biopsies, and the pelvitrainer.

He performed lysis of adhesions, intestinal sutures, biopsies, and staging of tumors, more than 200 hepatic biopsies and, above all, gynecological interventions.

At that time gynecological interventions were performed either by a median incision or by an incision of Pfannenstiel (Her- man J. Pfannenstiel, Gynaecologist at Kiel from 1907 -1909).

Based on his training both as a toolmaker and physician, his first inventions were to develop an electronic CO2 insufflator, a uterine manipulator and a tubal patency-testing device. He presented his works at the German, Austrian and Swiss gynecological meetings in the early 1960s. Palmer's work in France stimulated Semm's interests in gynecologic laparoscopy, leading to his invention of CO2 pneu-automatic insufflators [3] and pelviscopy [4] .

In **1984**, Semm described laparoscopic assistance vaginal hysterectomy (LAVH) in his book "Gynäkologische Laparoskopie" [5](Schattauer Publishing House, page 236). This "cookbook" for gynecological endoscopy, was translated into English and published by the American Yearbook Company.

In **1970**, the German surgeon **H. Hasson**[6] (Fig - 46) presented his technique and the relative instrument to access the peritoneum. His first publication concerning this technique appeared eight years later. In **1978**, he introduced an alternative method of trocar placement. He proposed a blunt mini-laparotomy which permits direct visualization of trocar entrance into the peritoneal cavity. A reusable device of similar design to a standard cannula but attached to an olive-shaped sleeve was developed by Hasson. This sleeve would slide up and down the shaft of the cannula and would form an airtight seal at the fascial opening. In addition, the sharp trocar was replaced by a blunt obturator. This cannula is held in place by the use of stay sutures passed through the fascial edges and attached to the body of the cannula. Pneumoperitoneum is then rapidly created. Hasson proposed its potential benefits to be the avoidance of blind insertion of the Veress needle and bladed trocar, prevention of visceral and vascular injuries, preperitoneal insufflation and gas embolism, guaranteed pneumoperitoneum, and a more anatomical repair of the abdominal wall. Since that time, many surgeons have made some modifications to first Hasson technique [7].

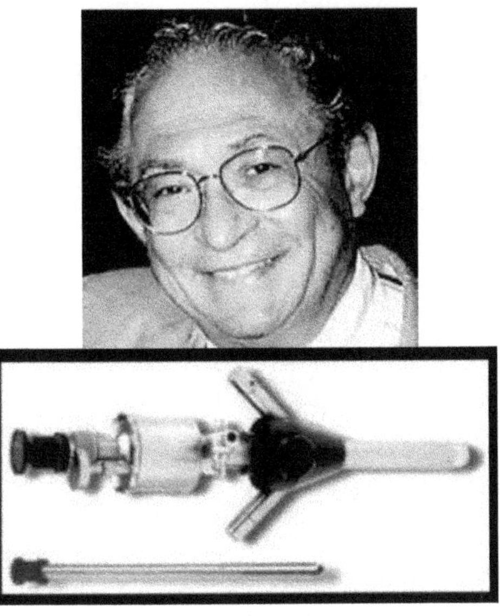

Fig – 46 Harrith Hasson

In **1977** First solid state camera was introduced [8]. This is the start of "video-laparoscopy". The final step was solid state camera technology of the 1980s that created the first wave of electronic digital cameras and portable video systems.

As video monitors improved the images on high definition displays, surgeons had the optical resolution they needed to discern the anatomic detail necessary to perform surgical operations of increasing complexity.

Their eye no longer locked onto the objective of the laparoscope held by one hand, surgeons could stand, view the operation on a video display, and perform standard operations using both hands. It was **Camran Nezhat**, (Fig – 47) considered the founding "father" of operative video-laparoscopy, who would use his visionary foresight and virtuoso surgical skill to bring this concept clamoring out of its dream-state and headlong into the realm of reality[9]. His papers were refused by established journals for years and, like Muhe and Semm, he was rewarded only with criticism, and ultimately a formal investigation, following which he was fully exonerated.[10]

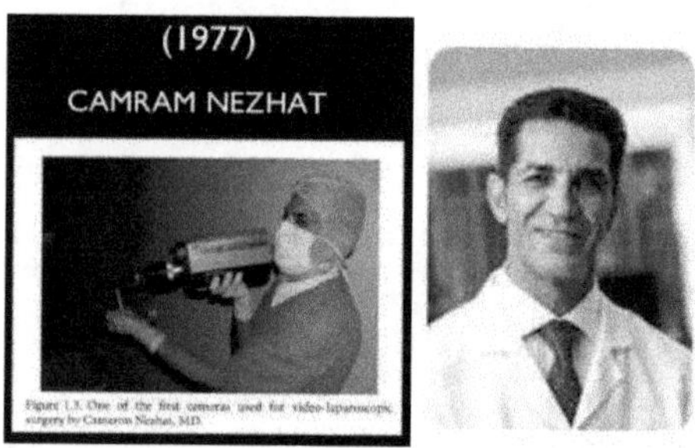

Fig – 47 Camran Nezhat born in Shahreza, Iran, American Nationality,Gynecologist.

In **1978 JR Dingfelder**[11] (Fig 48) developed the direct laparoscopic trocar insertion technique.He reported[12]and later it is described by Copeland etal in 1983,[12]but so far it has been used mainly by gynecologists.[13] According to Copeland et al,[12] the keys to a successful DTI are adequate wall relaxation, proper skin incision, and the use of a sharp trocar.[12]Currently, none of the available methods of entry into the peritoneal cavity for creation of pneumoperitoneum are free of complications. Each has its individual advantages and disadvantages and similar morbidity when performed by experienced operators with appropriate indications.[14]

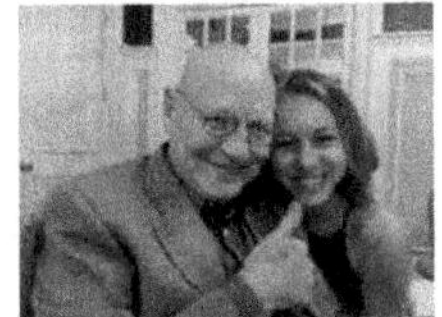

Fig – 48 JR Dingfelder

In **1979** another German surgeon, Dominic Frimberger had performed the first laparoscopic cholecystectomy on a **pig**, but the work was published many years later, the era of experimental laparoscopic cholecystectomy had begun.

In **1979**, the Robot Institute of America defined 'robot' as a machine comprised of four characteristics it is 'reprogrammable'; it is capable of manipulating materials, parts, and tools; it performs 'programmed' movements and it possesses the ability to perform more than one task.

In **1980** – **Patrick Steptoe** (Fig-49) from England started to perform laparoscopic procedures in the operating room under sterile conditions. Despite the negative attitude among his colleagues, Steptoe soon became one of the most innovative researchers in the field of abdominal endoscopy, particularly laparoscopic sterilization. In the late 1960s, Steptoe began working with Robert Edwards, an embryologist, and launched an in-vitro fertilization [15](I.V.F) project obtaining eggs by means of laparoscopy. Both researchers experienced years of frustration, disappointment, ethical and scientific criticism as well as a difficult relationship with the mass media. Finally, in July 1978, Louise Brown, the first test-tube baby, was born in England.

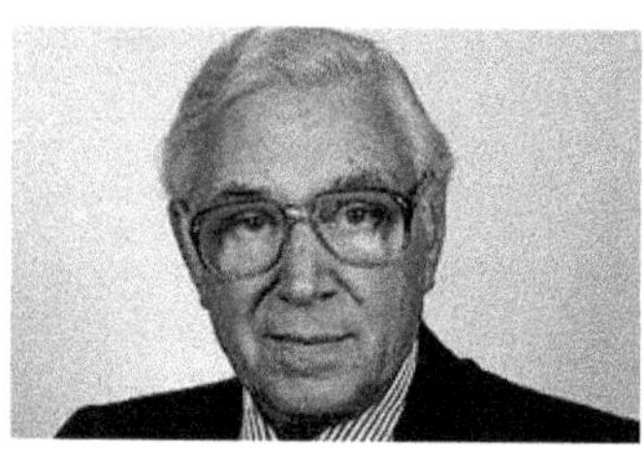

(Fig – 49) Patrick Steptoe (1978- 1988) Oxford, England.

The final step was solid state camera technology of the 1980s that created the first wave of electronic digital cameras and portable video systems.[16] As video monitors improved the images on high definition displays, surgeons had the optical resolution they needed to discern the anatomic detail necessary to perform surgical operations of increasing complexity. Their eye no longer locked onto the objective of the laparoscope held by one hand, surgeons could stand, view the operation on a video display, and perform standard operations using both hands

In **1983** the first laparoscopic appendectomy was performed [17]. Still in 1983 the British urologist J. E. A. Wickham coined the term "minimally invasive surgery" and in 1987 the first edition of the journal "Surgical Endoscopy" came out [18] .Barry J. McKerman, surgeon, and William B.Saye, gynaecologist, on June 22 1988 at Marietta in Georgia, performed the first cholecystectomy in the USA. In the same year it was performed by Eddie J. Reddick and Douglas O. Olsen in Nashville (Tennessee) (they also organised the first courses in the world in Laparoscopic Surgery), and subsequently at Los Angeles by Berci [19].

In **1985** Erich Mühe (Fig - 50) , a surgeon at the University of Boblingen in Germany, performed the first laparoscopic cholecystectomy on humans using a modified rectoscope as for access and with the insufflation with CO2. With his "Galloscope" he performed the first laparoscopic cholecystectomy [20,21]and he first documented laparoscopic cholecystectomy. In **1986** he presented the case to the German Society of Surgeons Congress in Munich, but the surgical community was not supportive. In the same year, he presented it to the Rhineland – Palatinate Surgical Society in Cologne, where he was again unsuccessful. He was practically unknown abroad: from 1965 to 1988 he published 342 articles, of which only 7% were in English.

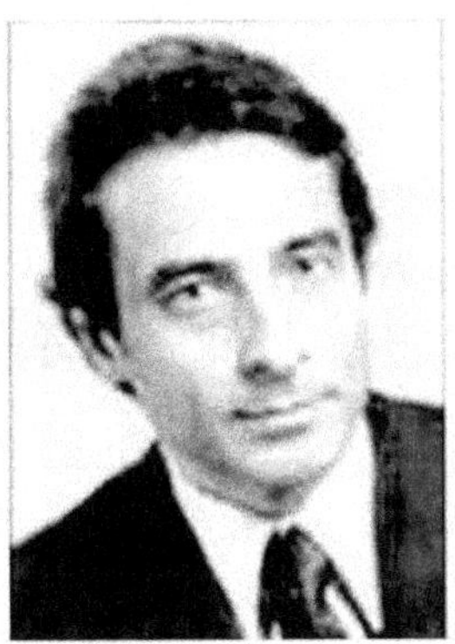

Fig -50 Erich Muhe.

In 1990 Muhe sent an article to the American Journal of Surgery on laparoscopic cholecystectomy: the article was rejected. In the same year, he met Dubois in Paris, and an argument almost erupted when the German surgeon claimed to have performed the first laparoscopic cholecystectomy. At the Second World Congress of the Society of American Gastrointestinal Endoscopic Surgery (SAGES) the question as to who was the first surgeon to perform a laparoscopic cholecystectomy was raised: the names Perissat, Reddick, Berci, Cuschieri, Dubois, and Mouret were proposed: Mühe was not mentioned. The official recognition by SAGES and therefore the whole scientific world finally occurred on March 26, 1999, in San Antonio, Texas, with the Annual Karl Storz Lecture in New Technology, it was awarded to Mühe. The title of the lecture was "The First Laparoscopic Cholecystectomy: Overcoming the Roadblocks on the Road to the Future". Although Mühe was accepted as the inventor, it was the French School that contributed the most to making laparoscopic cholecystectomy use common. In fact, many surgeons consider Mouret, Dubois, and Perissat the "Second French Revolution". In 1985, he in Boblingen, Germany, used Semm's instruments and technique to remove the first gallbladder in the world laparoscopically. In 1990, his article about the first laparoscopic cholecystectomies submitted to the *American Journal of Surgery* was rejected because of his difficulties with the English language. Finally, at the 109th German Surgical Society Congress (GSS) on April 21, 1992, his pioneering work in endoscopic surgery was recognized as one of the greatest original achievements of German medicine in recent history, and Muhe received the GSS Anniversary Award.[22]

In **1987** ,Translations into eight other languages followed. An extension of the book was recently published under the title "Endoskopische Abdominalchirurgie" (Editors: L. Mettler and K. Semm, Schattauer Publishing House, 2002.)

In **1986** video was adopted, after having been experimented since **1982**; video laparoscopic surgery (VLS) had arrived. In **1987 Philippe Mouret**, (Fig – 51) from Lyon performed the first cholecystectomy with 4 trocars on a patient with a gynecological disorder and gallstones. His laparoscopic procedure has significantly revolutionized general surgery. In the same period, Mühe had successfully performed 94 cholecystectomies, without the scientific world is aware. According to Philippe Mouret, the first cholecystectomy was performed quite naturally, without premeditation. The patient was a woman of about 50 years, suffering from painful pelvic adhesions, who had been referred to him for laparoscopic adhesiolysis. The patient also suffered from symptomatic gallbladder lithiasis, and had asked him if he would perform both operations at the same time. The operation schedule mentioned: "laparoscopy, gynecological adhesiolysis, and cholecystectomy."[23]

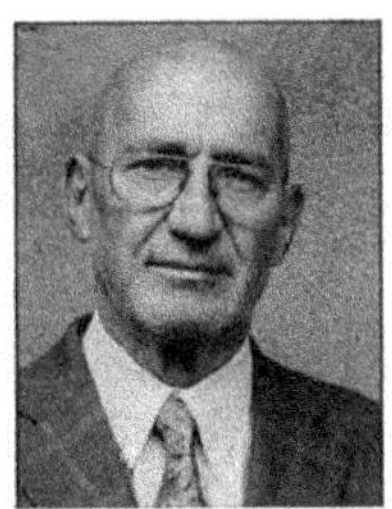

Fig – 51 Philippe Mouret, gynaecologist from Lyon.

In **1988 Donald P. Dubois** (Fig - 52) carried out the same intervention publishing his work the following year. In April 1989, Professor Jacques Perissat, whose presentation had not been accepted in the main program at the meeting of the Society of American Gastrointestinal Endoscopic Surgeons (SAGES) in Louisville, Kentucky displayed a videotape on laparoscopic cholecystectomy and described his technique in a remote booth of the exhibition area. This videotape quickly attracted a larger audience than did the lecturers in the main auditorium,[24] and marked the beginning of the worldwide revolution in laparoscopic surgery for general surgeons.[25]

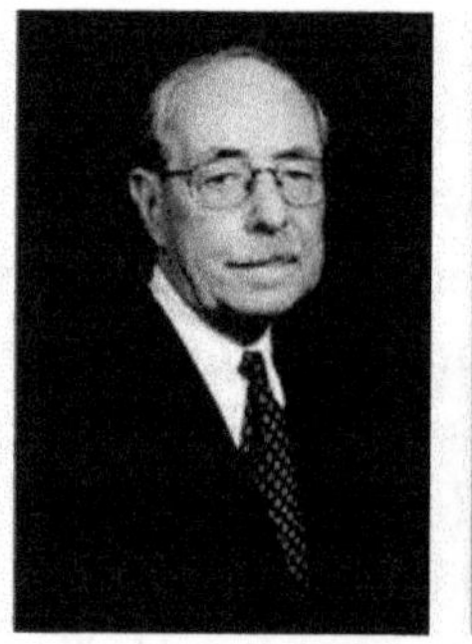

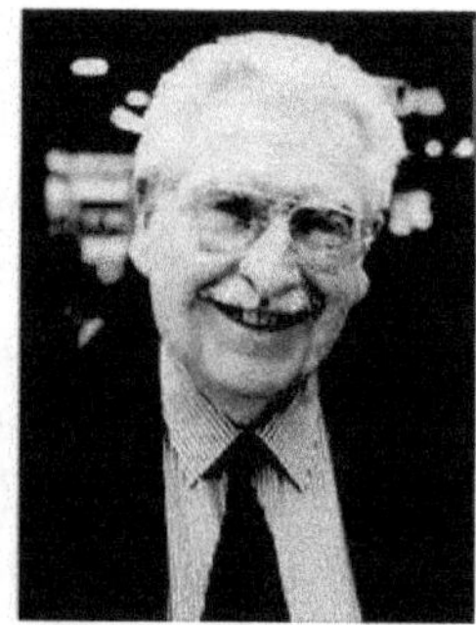

Fig - 52 Donald P. Dubois Figs – 53 Jaques Perissat.

During the same period in Bordeaux **Jacques Perissat** (Fig - 53), and in Dundee Alfred Cuschieri, performed the same operation. In **Moscow** in **1983**, D. Lukikev performed the first laparoscopic cholecystectomy which was censured by the Medical Academy. Still, in **1983** the British urologist **J. E. A. Wickham** coined the term "minimally invasive surgery" and in **1987** the first edition of the journal "Surgical Endoscopy" came out. From the point of view of the doctor-patient relationship, a quote from Perissat [26] is significant: "The laparoscopic revolution is particularly important because for the first time, surgery no longer involves any physical contact between the surgeon's hand and the patient. The very first surgical robot was used in an orthopedic surgical procedure on March 12, 1984, at the UBC Hospital in Vancouver.

Barry J. McKerman, the surgeon, and William B.Saye, on June 22, **1988**, at Marietta in Georgia, performed the first VLS cholecystectomy in the **USA**. In the same year, it was performed by Eddie J. Reddick and Douglas O. Olsen in Nashville (Tennessee) and organized **the first courses** in the world in Laparoscopic Surgery, and subsequently at Los Angeles by Berci .

Shortly thereafter the "laparoscopic revolution" broke out, and Semm's laparoscopic expertise was in great demand. His publications on the subject, translated into many languages, were read across the world by thousands of surgeons. Without Semm's input, the development of a "Laparoscopic Revolution," while perhaps inevitable would have been postponed by many years. A natural consequence was the development of new laparoscopic techniques for many other organs including the abdominal wall for repair of hernia, the colon, the stomach, the esophagus, the kidney, the spleen, the bladder, the adrenal gland, the pancreas, the liver, the common bile duct, the aorta, and other intrathoracic structures. In **1987** Ger reported first laparoscopic repair of inguinal hernia using prototype stapler.In January **1989**, Harry Reich (Fig -54) described first laparoscopic hysterectomy using bipolar desiccation at pennsylvania; later he demonstrated staples and finally sutures for laparoscopic hysterectomy.By the **1990**s nearly all operations in every major speciality could be done using laparoscopy and minimally invasive methods ,a true revolution in surgery.

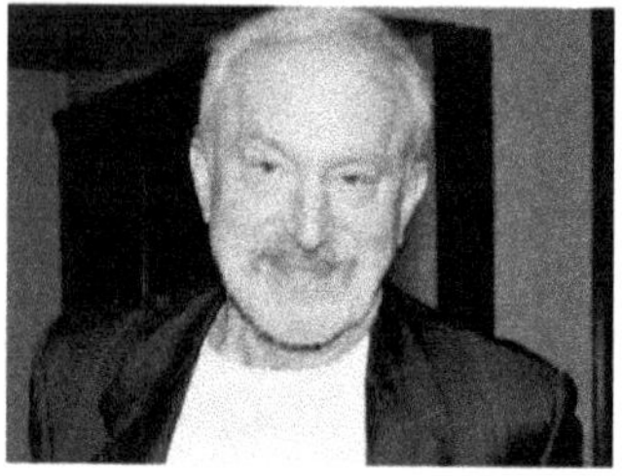

Fig – 54 Harry Reich

In **1994** A **robotic arm** (Fig -55) was designed to hold the laparoscope camera and instruments with the goal of improving safety, reducing the need of skilled camera operator, resource utilization and improving efficiency and versatility for the surgeon. Current robotics on the market include "Zeus" originally designed by Computer Motion (which merged with Intuitive Surgical in 2003), and the "da Vinci" robot that is currently on the market by Intuitive Surgical [27]. They have not yet been designed and programed to perform all minimally invasive procedures and therefore will not be replacing the surgeon any time soon.The feasibility of robotic-assisted surgery has been examined for a variety of laparoscopic procedures. In 2001, Cadiére and colleagues published a robotic-assisted laparoscopic surgery series using the Da Vinci system (Intuitive Surgical), including three inguinal hernia repairs.[28]Although the robotic articulating instruments facilitated dissection in a variety of procedures, one system limitation noted was the narrow field of vision provided by the three-dimensional optical system. Engelberger started the first commercial company to make robots called 'Unimation' (universal automation). Devol wrote the necessary patents. Their first robot was called the 'Unimate'. This resulted in Engelberger being called the 'father of robotics.'

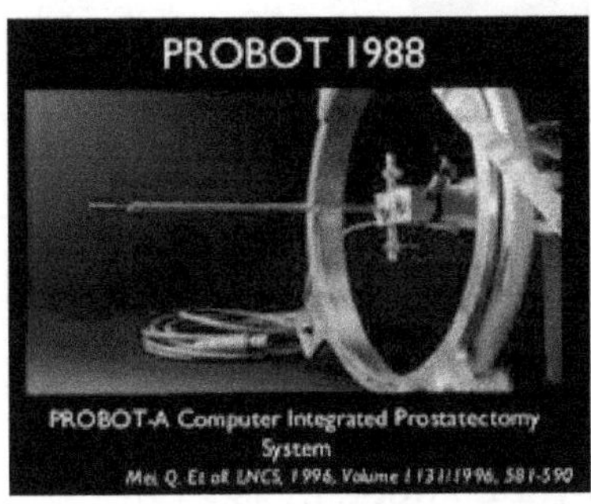

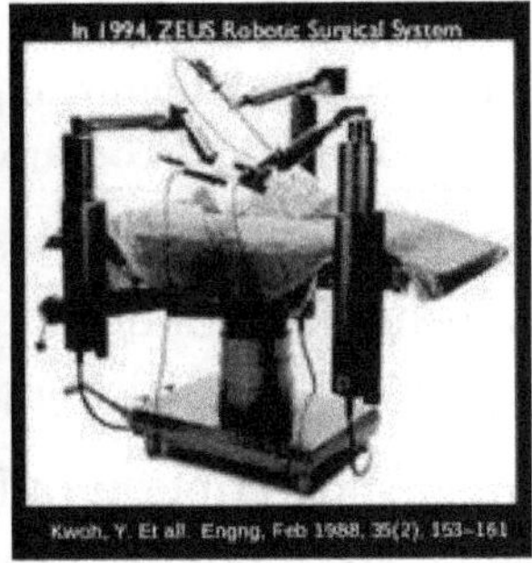

Fig – 55 Robotic arm

In **1996** First live broadcast of laparoscopic surgery via the Internet. (Robotic Telesurgery). After preparatory cases using porcine models, Dr. Marescaux performed a robotic minimally invasive cholecystectomy between New York City and his patient, a 68-year-old woman in Strasbourg, France [29].In addition, the first transnational telesurgery was performed in 2001 on a patient in France while the operating surgeon was 6.500 km away in New York.[30]

First **Robotic** Laparoscopic surgery done by Dan Stoianovici (Fig-56) in 1993 .He lead to the use of this device for brachytherapy [31]. Robotic Surgery Food and Drug Administration approved in 2000.

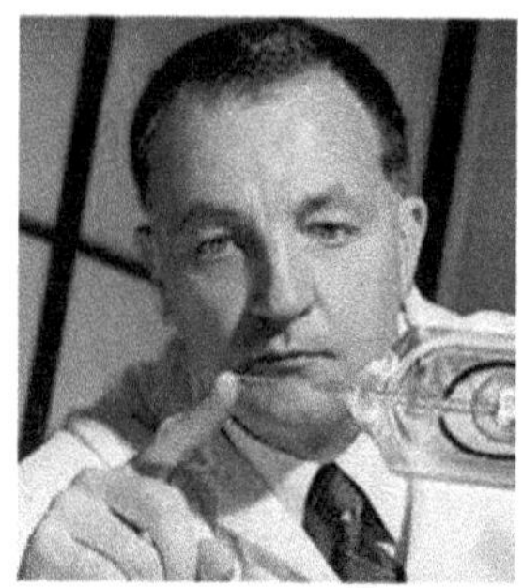

Fig-56.Dan Stoianovici, Professor of Urology, Urology Robotics Program Johns Hopkins Medicine.

In **2004** the first work on NOTES (Natural Orifice Transluminal Endoscopic Surgery) was published: the hepatic trans-gastric biopsy was among the first surgeries

The first description of **laparoscopic pancreatoduodenectomy** (LPD) done in 1994 by Gagner and Pomp (Fig -57)

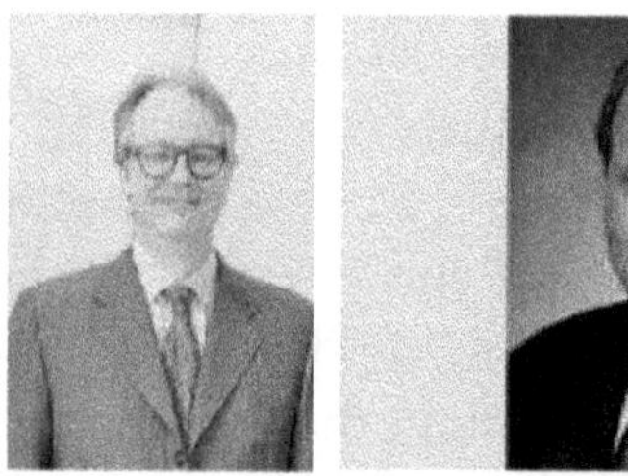

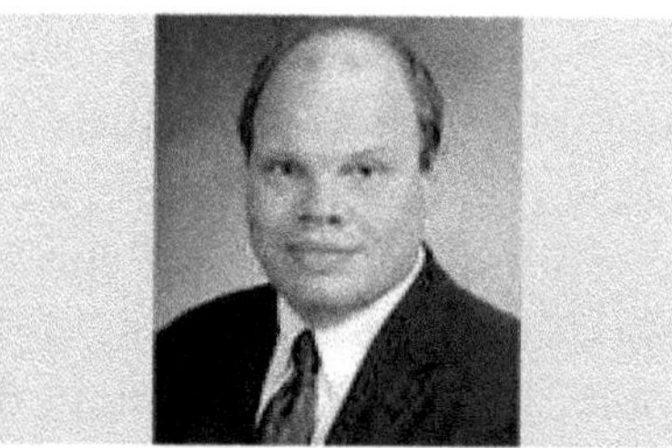

Fig – 57 .Dr. Michel Gagner and Pomp, Chief of GI Metabolic and Bariatric Surgery.

Cleveland Clinic Foundation Ohio, New York, U.S .

Dr.C.Palanivelu(Fig - 58) ,India - Recorded the Laparoscopic Whipple operation (LPD) for cancer Pancreas first to perform and completed first time in the world,2007 with largest series published in the world.

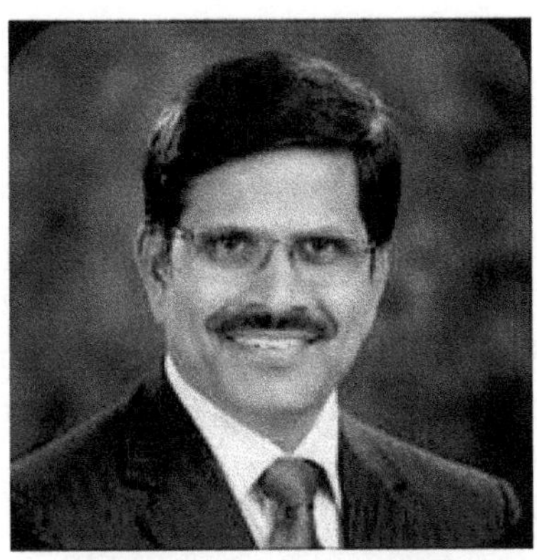

Fig – 58. Dr.C.Palanivelu ,India.

He recorded first as "The standard technique"with Palanivelu prone technique for thoracic laparoscopic Oesophagectomy.He made a unique Hydatid trocar system for Hydatid cyst Liver excision. He is the first Indian surgeon did laparoscopic mesh repair for Incisional Hernia with primary closure of the defect.

Palanivelu[32] and Zornig [33] have shown hybrid approach success in cholecystectomies, while the combination of miniature surgical robots and/or transabdominal magnet devices with flexible endoscopic instruments is a rapidly developing modification with promising perspectives.

The first documented procedures Single incision laparoscopy (**SILS**) of significance occurred in the late **1990s**. The first described single-port laparoscopy (SPL) procedure was a **gall bladder** removal in **1997**.Earliest evidence of N.O.T.E.S can be traced to **1901** when Dimitri Oskarovich Ott performed endoscopic examination of the peritoneal cavity through the vagina. The procedure then was termed "ventroscopy".[34]

In **2004** the first work on NOTES (Natural Orifice Transluminal Endoscopic Surgery)[35][36] was published: the hepatic trans-gastric biopsy was among the first surgeries [37].On June 25, **2007** Swanstrom (Fig – 59) and colleagues reported the first human transgastric cholecystectomy.

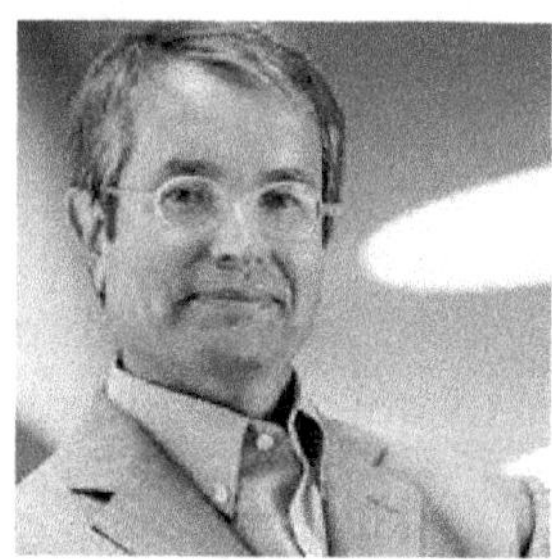

Fig – 59 .Lee Swanstrom - NOTES Cholecystectom Institute of Image-Guided Surgery (IHU Strasbourg, France)

NOTES Originally described in animals by researchers at Johns Hopkins University (Dr Anthony Kalloo et al). Transgastric appendectomy in humans in India reported by Dr.G.V.Rao and Dr. D.N. Reddy[38] [39](Fig - 60)

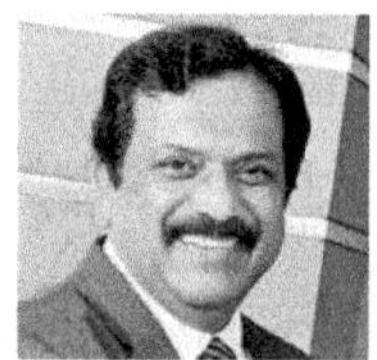

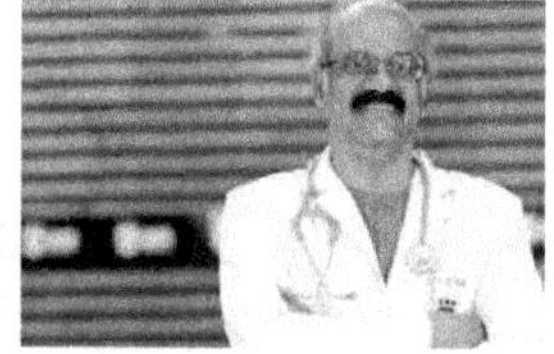

Fig – 60.Dr.G.V Rao & Dr. D.Nageshwar Reddy

Hyderabad, India. NOTES –Appendicectomy

Successful studies of N.OT.E.S in Humans with a tabular compilation[40].

Successful N.O.T.E.S in humans.

Author	Year	Procedure	Number of patients
Palanivelu et al[14,42]	2009	TV cholecystectomy	6
	2008	TV appendicectomy	1/6
Auyang et al[52]	2009	TG hybrid cholecystectomy	4
Vitale et al[54]	2009	TG drainage of pancreatic abcess	28
Zorrón et al[12,13,40]	2008	TV peritoneoscopy + liver, diaphragm, ovary biopsy	1
	2008	TV cholecystectomy	4
	2007	TV cholecystectomy	1
Hazey et al[55]	2008	TG peritoneoscopy	10
Marks et al[56]	2007	PEG rescue, TG peritoneoscopy	1
Rao and Reddy[43]	2006	TG appendicectomy	1

TV – transvaginal; TG – transgastric.

Though N.O.T.E.S is still being developed and trialed, other alternatives using hybrid approaches such as natural orifice tran-sumbilical surgery (NOTUS) have shown promise. Nguyen etal [41,42] have shown success at performing sleeve gastrectomy and chole-cystectomy in human model using NOTUS.Whether these procedures compete against or complement N.O.T.E.S in the future needs to be seen.With patient choice taking precedence in the western world,N.O.T.E.S may be the cosmetic surgery of the future.Hence,there maybe pressure on the surgeons to develop this technique which has a steep learning curve. N.O.T.E.S has a future which is engulfed in the mist of unknown outcomes; only time will serve as the best judge.

FUTURE

A number of new approaches have already evolved, some even aggressively marketed, even though they have not yet been sufficiently established or their impact adequately studied. It should be in the interest of our specialty to develop objective guidance to such efforts and determine the goals and possible benefit/risk analysis in the context of health economics before pushing too hard into a respective direction.

1.Robotic vs laparoscopic surgery

The bulkiness of the robotic machine as such, the fact that the surgeon's assistants at the table only see a 2-dimensional image, the cost and some recent data from other specialties about increased rates of nerve injury appear as distinct disadvantages and warrant a more objective evaluation in the near future[43,44].

2.Number of incisions

Single port laparoscopic surgery or NOTES . They were once perceived to be the ultimate goal of minimally invasive surgery.However, despite enthusiasm, it appears that single port surgeries offer no advantage compared to conventional laparoscopic surgery[45,46].

3.Telesurgery.

Also known as remote surgery. Will be instrumental if astronauts are to travel to Mars or other planets—performing surgical procedures in space. Despite the introduction of numerous telesurgical innovations since 2001, only a single randomized controlled telesurgery trial of percutaneous access of the kidney with a remote center of motion active robotic device (PAKY-RCM) exists to date[47]. In addition to the need for further optimization of visual display, latency time, and haptic feedback technology, further randomized controlled trials should be performed to lead to the innovations' successful clinical translation [48,49].

Future developments will probably focus on the improvement of intraoperative imaging techniques, improved tactile feedback through the so-called ‘endohand’,[50] navigation,[51] and robotic assista

A veritable explosion of new tools occurred with the hundreds of new surgical procedures which were developed in the 19th century and first decades of the 20th century. New materials, such as stainless steel, chrome, titanium and vanadium were available for the manufacturing of these instruments. Precision instruments for microsurgery in neurosurgery, ophthalmology and otology were possible and, in the second half of the 20th century, energy-based instruments were first developed, such as electrocauteries, ultrasound and electric scalpels, surgical tools for endoscopic surgery, and finally, surgical robots. Close collaborations between industry and surgeons were at the forefront of developing sophisticated instrumentation and technology according to the true needs in the operative field. Multiple aspects of various surgical procedure steps were optimized by introduction of new devices and equiment such as energy and sealing devices, staplers, and clipappliers [52].

What is the next evolutionary step? Clarice Powers suggested that, “futuristic surgical interventions will move from minimally invasive techniques to non-invasive techniques. Concepts such as virtual reality, virtual imaging, robotics, and remote surgical interventions may well be the norm in operating rooms of the next decade”[53]. From her viewpoint in 1990, Powers had the right idea. While virtual reality still lives in imagination, robotics have made their way into the operating room.

In the future, laparoscopic surgery will definitely continue to develop based on the technically updated advancements and new surgeries will become possible which were kept previously in the list of relative indications for difficult possibility. The journey is continuous to explore the finest corners of the evidence based science and technology for the maximum benefit of the patients and their early recovery.

Referrences

1. Contribution on the method of utero-tubal perturbation - FIKENTSCHER R, SEMM K,Geburtshilfe Frauenheilkd. 1955 Apr; 15(4):313-22.
2. (Courtesy of Monika Bals-Pratsch MD, Zentrum für Gyn.kologie, Universit.t Regensburg, Germany)
3. Raoul Palmer, World War II, and transabdominal coelioscopy. Laparoscopy extends into gynecology.,Litynski GS.JSLS. 1997 Jul-Sep; 1(3):289-92.
4. Semm K. Pelviscopy – operative guidelines. UFK Kiel, Kiel:1992
5. Semm K. *Gynäkologische Laparoskopie*. Stuttgart: Schattauer Publishing House; 1984.
6. Hasson HM. Open laparoscopy vs. closed laparoscopy: a comparison of complication rates. Adv Plan Parent 1978;13:41-50.
7. Akush Ginekol (Sofiia),2015;54(4):52-6.OPEN LAPAROSCOPY--A MODIFIED HASSON TECHNIQUE - Article in Bulgarian

8. 2005 Presidential Address - *Nezhat C,JSLS. 2005 Oct-Dec; 9(4):370-5*

9. Society of laparoscopic & Robotic surgeons,Chapter 22 – Nazhat & Rise of Advanced Operative Video Laoparoscopy,Chaper by Barbara Page

10. Nezhat C, Page B. Let There Be Light: an Historical Analysis of Endoscopy's Ascension since Antiquity. January 2008.

11. Dingfelder JR. Direct laparoscopic trocar insertion without prior pneumoperitoneum. *J Reprod Med.* 1978;21:45–47

12. Copeland C, Wing R, Huka JF. Direct trocar insertion at laparoscopy: an evaluation. *Obstet Gynecol.* 1983;62:665–669

13. Byron JW, Fusjiyoshi CA, Miyazawa K. Evaluation of direc trocar insertion technique at laparoscopy. *Obstet Gynecol.* 1989;74:423–425

14. Woolcott R. The safety of laparoscopy performed by direct trocar insertion and carbon dioxide insufflation under vision. *Aust N Z J Obstet Gynaecol.* 1997;37(2):216–219

15. Edwards R, Steptoe PC.A *Matter of Life. The Story of a Medical Breakthrough.* London: Hutchinson Publishers; 1980

16. Fossum ER. Camera-on-achip: Technology transfer from Saturn to your cell phone. Technology Innovation. 2013; 15(3):197-209.

17. Lytinski GC. Endoscopic Surgery: The History, The Pioneers. Word J Surg 1999;23:745-753.

18. Lytinski GS. Highlights in the history of laparoscopy. Frankfurt, Verlag Pubs 1996.

19. Morgenstern L. George Berci past, present and future. Surg Endosc 2006;20:410-411.

20. Muhe E. Die erste Cholecystectomie durch das Laparoskop. Langenbecks Arch Chir. 1986;**369**:804.

21. Muhe E. Laparoscopic cholecystectomy - late results. Langenbecks Arch Chir. 1991;**Suppl**:416–423.

22. Reynolds W., Jr The first laparoscopic cholecystectomy. *JSLS*. 2001;5:89–94

23. Mouret P. How I developed laparoscopic cholecystectomy. *Ann Acad Med Singapore*. 1996;25:744–747

24. Dent TL. Framework for the future. The 1997 Gerald Marks Lecture. Society of American Gastrointestinal Endoscopic Surgeons (SAGES). March 22, 1997. *Surg Endosc*. 1997;11:975–978

25. Himal HS. Minimally invasive (laparoscopic) surgery. *Surg Endosc*. 2002;16:1647–1652

26. Perissat J. Laparoscopic Surgery: a pioneer's point of view. World J Surg 1999;23:863-868

27. Culjat, Martin, Rahul Singh, and Hua Lee. Medical Devices Surgical and Imageguided Technologies. Hoboken, N.J.: John Wiley & Sons, 2012. 29-96.

28. Cadiére GB, Himpens J, Germay O, et al. Feasibility of robotic laparoscopic surgery: 146 cases. World J Surg 2001; 25: 1467–77

29. Marescaux J, Leroy J, Rubino F, et al. Transcontinental robot-assisted remote telesurgery: feasibility and potential applications. *Ann Surg*. 2002;235:487–492.

30. Marescaux J, Leroy J, Gagner M, et al. Transatlantic robot-assisted telesurgery. *Nature*.

31. Fichtinger G, Burdette EC, Tanacs A, Patriciu A, Mazilu D, Whitcomb LL, et al. Robotically assisted prostate brachytherapy with transrectal ultrasound guidance--Phantom experiments. *Brachytherapy*. 2006;5:14–26.

32. Palanivelu C, Rajan PS, Rangarajan M, Parthasarathi R, Senthilnathan P,Praveenraj P. Transumbilical flexible endoscopic cholecystectomy in humans:first feasibility study using a hybrid technique.Endoscopy2008;40:428–31.

33. Zornig C, Mofid H, Emmermann A, Alm M, von Waldenfels HA, Felixmu ̈ller C.Scarless cholecystectomy with combined

transvaginal and transumbilicalapproach in a series of 20 patients.Surg Endosc2008;22:1427–9.

34. M.F. McGee, M.J. Rosen, J. Marks,A primer on natural orifice translumenal endoscopic surgery: building a new paradigm,Surg Innov, 13 (2006), pp. 86-93

35. Kalloo AN, Singh VK, Jagannath SB, Niiyama H, Hill SL, Vaughn CA, Magee CA, Kantsevoy SV. Flexible transgastric peritoneoscopy: a novel approach to diagnostic and therapeutic interventions in the peritoneal cavity. Gastrointest Endosc 2004;60:114-117.

36. Tsao AK., Averch TD. The history of NOTES. J Endourol 2009;23:727-731.

37. Steele K, Schweitzer MA, Lyn-Sue J, Kantsevoy SV. Flexible transgastric peritoneoscopy and liver biopsy: a feasibility study in human beings (with videos). Gastrointest Endosc 2008;68:61-6.

38. Tropicalgastro, Quarterly Reviews, NOTES: A review- Magnus Jayaraj Mansard, D Nageshwar Reddy, G Venkat Rao

39. NOTES: human experience,May 2008,Gastrointestinal Endoscopy Clinics of North America 18(2):361-70;

40. Natural orifice translumenal endoscopic surgery (N.O.T.E.S)P.N. Nesargikara,*, S.S. JaunoobaKeele School of Medicine and University Hospital of North Staffordshire, UKbWorcestershire Royal Hospital, UK.

41. Nguyen NT, Reavis KM, Hinojosa MW, Smith BR, Wilson SE. Laparoscopictransumbilical sleeve gastrectomy without visible abdominal scars.Surg ObesRelat Dis2009;5:275–7.

42. Nguyen NT, Reavis KM, Hinojosa MW, Smith BR, Wilson SE. Laparoscopictransumbilical cholecystectomy without visible abdominal scars.J GastrointestSurg2008

43. Robotically assisted vs laparoscopic hysterectomy among women with benign gynecologic disease.,Wright JD, Ananth CV, Lewin SN, Burke WM, Lu YS, Neugut AI, Herzog TJ, Hershman DL,JAMA. 2013 Feb 20; 309(7):689-98.

44. Prospective evaluation with standardised criteria for postoperative complications after robotic-assisted laparoscopic radical prostatectomy.,*Novara G, Ficarra V, D'Elia C, Secco S, Cavalleri S, Artibani W,Eur Urol. 2010 Mar; 57(3):363-70.*

45. Fung AK, Aly EH. Systematic review of single-incision laparoscopic colonic surgery. Br J Surg. 2012;**99**:1353–1364.

46. Kanakala V, Borowski DW, Agarwal AK, Tabaqchali MA, Garg DK, Gill TS. Comparative study of safety and outcomes of single-port access versus conventional laparoscopic colorectal surgery. Tech Coloproctol. 2012;**16**:423–428.

47. Telemedicine in surgery: what are the opportunities and hurdles to realising the potential? Raison N, Khan MS, Challacombe B. *Curr Urol Rep.* 2015;16:43.

48. Telesurgery is promising but still need proof through prospective comparative studies. Stark M, Morales ER, Gidaro S. *J Gynecol Oncol.* 2012;23:134–135.

49. A new telesurgical platform--preliminary clinical results. Stark M, Pomati S, D'Ambrosio A, Giraudi F, Gidaro S. *Minim Invasive Ther Allied Technol.* 2015;24:31–36.

50. Cuschieri A. Neue Technologien in der laparoskopischen Chirurgie. Chirurg 2001; 72: 252–60

51. Van der Peet DL, Berends FJ, Klinkenberg-Knol EC, Cuesta MA. Endoscopic treatment of benign esophageal tumors. Surg Endosc 2001; 15: 1489

52. World J Gastroenterol. 2014 Nov 7; 20(41): 15119–15124. Evolution and future of laparoscopic colorectal surgery

53. Powers, Clarice J. "A Brief History of Endoscopy." Seminars in Perioperative Nursing 2.3 (1993): 129-32.

7. Pre-peritoneal Space & Hernia Surgery

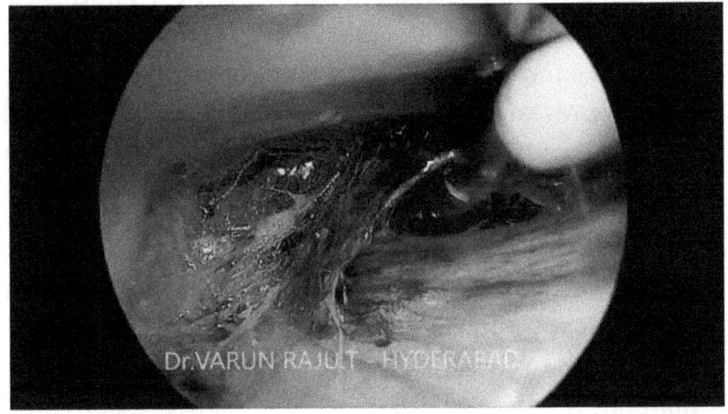

Preperitoneal (preperitoneal) space is the space between the peritoneum and transversalis fascia.

In 1919 La Roque in America had described an approach through the routine inguinal

incision, the extraperitoneal space being entered through a small muscle-splitting incision about an inch above the internal ring.

The posterior preperitoneal approach became established in the **1920s-1960s**, along with the use of prostheses. The tension free repair has now become the treatment of choice particularly the Lichtenstein repair is still the first recommended operation for inguinal hernia.

Bogros[1] (**1786-1825**) in 1823 described his preperitoneal space which continues into the suprapubic space of Retzius. He described a triangular space in the iliac region between the iliac fascia, transversalis fascia, and parietal peritoneum. In the modern concept, this space lies between the peritoneum and posterior lamina of the transversalis fascia. In **1858**, Retzius described the homonymous space, situated anterior and lateral to the urinary bladder (prevesical space). In **1975**, Fowler reported that the preperitoneal fascia of the groin is distinct from the transversalis fascia.

Annandale[2] initiated anterior preperitoneal repair. Cheatle[3] demonstrated the median posterior preperitoneal approach, resurrected by Henry [4] modified the Cheatle-Henry procedure by using a unilateral oblique incision in the rectus sheath and underlying transversalis fascia with medial retraction of the rectus muscle.

Stoppa et al., beginning in 1965, performed giant prosthetic reinforcement of the visceral sac, covering Fruchaud's myopectineal orifice preperitoneally with extensive overlap. They used a posterior approach to avoid scarring in recurrent cases and to allow the exposure of large, bilateral, inguinal, and femoral sacs[5], proposed a unilateral version.

Preperitoneal approaches to the repair of primary, bilateral, recurrent, inguinal, and femoral herniae, the most common abdominal protrusions, now dominate techniques of repair. The idea of repairing a groin hernia from the posterior side, in a preperitoneal position, was already suggested in the 18th century, namely.U.C.Bates (1875) in **1913** made analogous propositions. However it got definitely accepted after the proposal of George La Roque [6](1976-1934) in **1919** . A totally extraperitoneal approach was first executed by Cheatle[7] in **1920**, as a radical operation for cure of both inguinal and femoral herniae via a lower mid abdominal preperitoneal approach, an incision he preferred for such cure over a Pfannenstiel incision. His operation never seems to have become popular despite a plea for it by Williams (1938).

Sir Leanthal Cheatle used a vertical rectus-splitting incision, but later (1921) preferred a Pfannenstiel; he mobilised and isolated the processus vaginalis from the vas and vessels and then divided it; the distal end was either excised or ligated as low as possible. He carried out no repair and ended by examining the opposite side through the same incision; no follow-up of his series was ever published.

Henry[8] (1936) re described Cheatle's approach, via a midline incision, at first recommending it for femoral and then for inguinal herniae (1936). In the inguinal case he repaired the internal ring by suturing the edges of the transversalis fascia firmly round the cord.The extraperitoneal approach and midline incision were also advocated by Jennings[9] and his associates (1942). However, Jennings later returned to the orthodox method as he found that the inability to repair anything other than the transversalis fascia was unsatisfactory in large indirect herniae (Jennings 1960).

The use of the Rectus Sheath approach for femoral herniae by Peter G. McEvedy[10] (1950)

re-awakened interest in this approach to inguinal herniae either through an oblique incision (McEvedy 1958) or through a transverse incision three inches above the inguinal ligament Nyhus[11], Condon and Harkins, 1960; Smith, 1962. However, it seems that while there are certain advantages in the extraperitoneal approach, the disadvantages preclude its routine use[12][13][14].

In **1969** Rene Stoppa[15] (Fig-61) from Amiens developed a technique of GPRVS (giant prosthetic reinforcement of the visceral sac). René Stoppa was markedly in Xuenced by his lengthy exposure to, and formative years in, anatomy.The professional and academic endeavors of Professor Stoppa were dedicated to general surgery, with an early orientation toward gastro-intestinal surgery and a defenite tendency toward surgery of the abdominal wall[16].

In 1965, he designed,developed, and disseminated a personally developed technique in groin hernia repair - wrapping of the vis- ceral (hernial) sac with a large synthetic sheet through a midline pre-peritoneal approach applicable to multi- ple recurrent groin hernias and incisional hernias. Several thousand cases of such hernias have been the subject of French and international publications.

René Stoppa authored more than 500 publications in French and international journals, produced twelve surgical Wlms, and organized or presided over several national and international events.

Gifted with a keen sense of curiosity, Professor Stoppa always cultivated an interest in surgical innovations for which he kept a largely open eye and mind.

This technique was supposed to be applied to large, complicated and bilateral inguinal hernias and consisted on implanting a large polyester mesh in preperitoneal connective tissue between the peritoneum and fascia transversalis. The incision of choice for preperitoneal access was a low midline incision and the mesh need not to be fixed with sutures due to its size and intraabdominal pressure maintaining it in situ.

Laparoscopic repair of groin protrusions began in 1982 by Ger[17] In 1992, Arregui [18]et al. and Dion and Morin[19] reported on their transabdominal preperitoneal (TAPP) approach. To avoid intraperitoneal complications, Dulucq [20] recommended a totally extraperitoneal (TEP) approach.

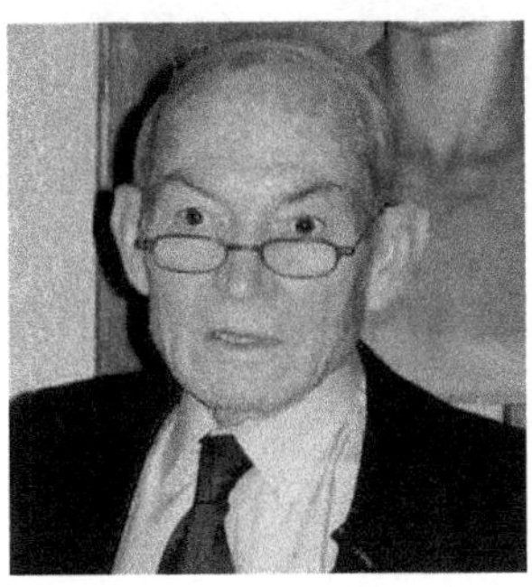

Fig –61 Professor René Stoppa (1921–2006),French Algeria.France.

In the **1970**'s Lloyd Nyhus (Fig - 62), from the University of Illinois and Cook County Hospital in Chicago and Robert Condon from the University of

Wisconsin in Madison popularized the pre-peritoneal approach for repair of all inguinal and femoral hernias. Unlike in the Stoppa method the incision was made above the inguinal ligament.

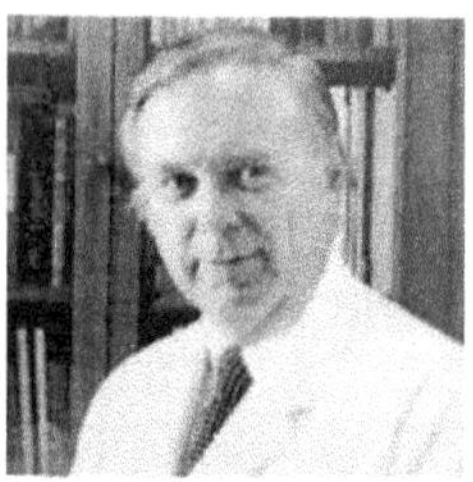

Fig – 62 - Lloyd Nyhus, Chicago,U.S

A similar incision was used also for a preperitoneal placement of a sutureless mesh by Robert Kugel)Fig – 63) from Olimipia in his technique described in **1999** and coined Kugel Hernia Patch .

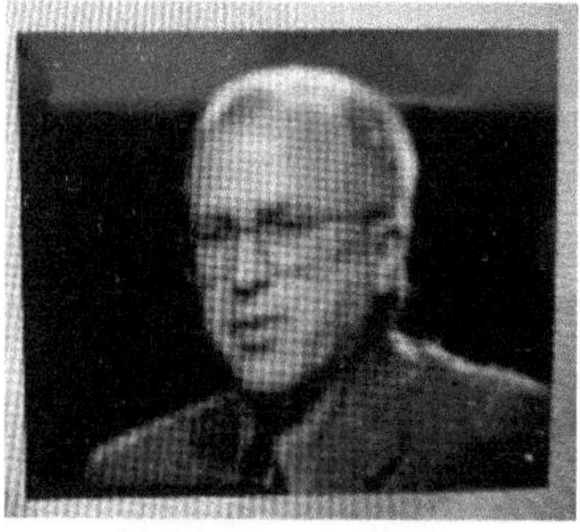

Fig – 63.Robert Kugel from Olimipia, Turek County, Greater Poland.

Jean Rives(Fig 64) and Jean-Henri Alexandre, both anatomists and surgeons, have been early educated since **1958–1960** in the use of prosthetic material in incisional hernia surgery by Pr Bourgeon at the French University of Algiers, about the same period as Usher **(1958)** and Koontz first publications on that topic.

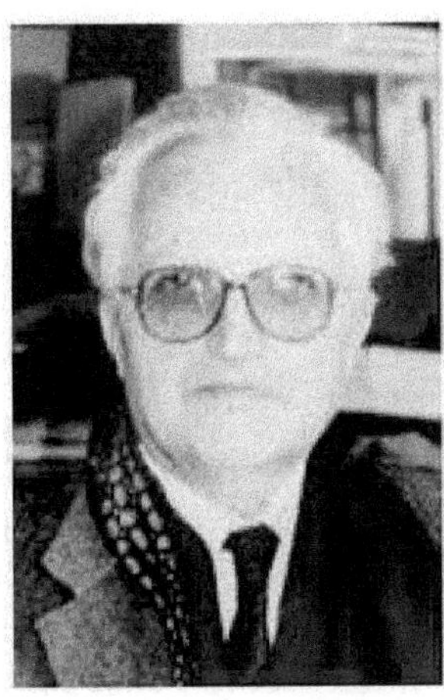

Fig – 64 .Jean Rives

Referrences

1. BOGROS (Essai sur l'anatomie chirurgical de la region iliac et description d'un nouveau procede pour faire la ligature des arteries epigastric et iliaque externe. Th. Paris, no. 153. A Paris, de l'imprimerie de Didot le Jeune, imprimeur de la Faculte de Medicine, rue des Macons, Sorbonne no. 13, 1823.

2. Edinb Med J 21:1087-1091, 1876.

3. Br Med J 2:68-69, 1920, Br Med J 2:1025-1026, 1921.

4. Lancet 1:531-533, 1936. McEvedy (Ann R Coll Surg Engl 7:484-496, 1950.

5. Rev Med Picardie 1:46-46, 1972). Wantz (Surg Gynecol Obstet, 169:408-417, 1989.

6. LA RoQuE, G. P. (1924): An Improved Method of Removing Hernia from Within, Ann. Surg., 79, 375. LA RoQUE, G. P. (1932): The Intra-Abdominal Method of Removing Inguinal and Femoral Hernia, Arch. Surg., 24, 189.

7. CHEATLE,G. L. (1920): An Operation for the Radical Cure of Inguinal and Femoral Herniae, Brit. med. J., ii, 68. CHEATLE, G. L. (1921): An Operation for Inguinal Hernia, Brit. med. J., ii, 1025.

8. HENRY, A. K. (1936(a)):, Proc. roy. Soc. Med., 30, 534. HENRY, A. K. (1936(b)): Operation for Femoral Hernia by a Midline Extra-Peritoneal Approach, Lancet, iL 531.

9. JENNINGS, W. K., ANSON, B. J., and WRIGHT, R. R. (1942): A New Method of Repair for Indirect Inguinal Hernia Considered in Reference to Parietal Anatomy, Surg. Gynec. Obstet., 74, 697. JENNINGS, W. K. (1960): Amer. J. Surg., 100, 243

10. McEVEDY, P. G. (1950): Femoral Hernia, Ann. roy. Coll. Surg. Engl., 7, 484. MCEVEDY, B. V. (1958): Inguinal Hernia; the Rectus Sheath Approach, W.Ajr. Med. J., 7, 106.

11. NyHus, L. M., CONDON, R. E., and HARKiss, H. N. (1960): Clinical Experience with Pre-Peritoneal Hernial Repair of all Types of Hernia of the Groin, Amer. J. Surg., 100, 234.

12. SMITH, A. N. (1962): A Rectus Sheath Extra-perntoneal Operation for Recurrent Inguinal Hernia, J. roy. Coll. Surg. Edinb., 7, 195.

13. WILLIAMS, C. (1938): The Advantages of the Abdominal Approach to Inguinal Hernia, Ann. Surg., 107, 917.

14. THE INTERNAL APPROACH FOR INGUINAL HERNIAE BRIAN V. MCEVEDY, M.CH., F.R.C.S. The Royal Victoria Infirmary, Newcastle-upon-Tyne ,POSTORAD. MED. J. (1966), 42, 548.

15. Stoppa R, Quintyn M. Les deficiences de la paroi abdominale chez le subject age: colloque avec le practicien. Sem Hosp 1969;45:2182.

16. Hernia (2007) 11:1–3 ,OBITUARY,René Stoppa (1921–2006)-Pierre Verhaeghe · Robert Bendavid

17. Ger; Ann R Coll Surg Engl 64:342-344, 1982.

18. Surg Laparosc Endosc 2:53-58, 1992.

19. Can J Surg 35:209-212, 1992.

20. Cahiers Chir 79:15-16, 1991.

8.Fascia Transversalis and Hernia Surgery

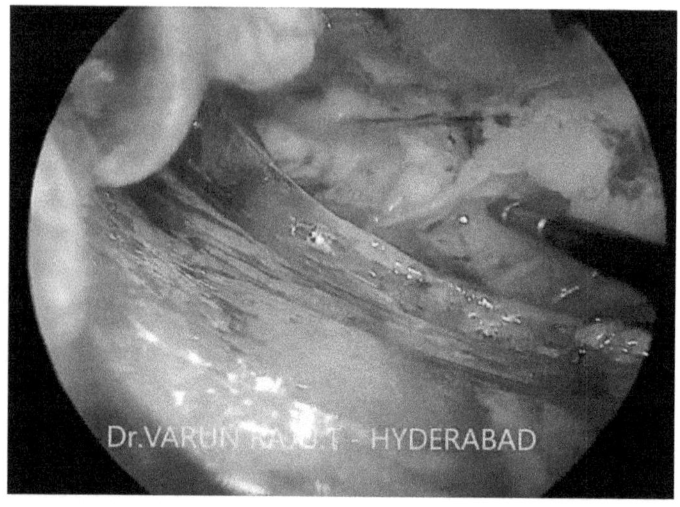

The strengthening of the transversalis fascia with prosthetic material, be it via

an external or internal approach, got boosted by new knowledge about the aetiology of

direct inguinal hernias. A deficiency in collagen, resulting from impairment of proline

and lysine hydroxylation proved to be the cause of weakening of this fascia, which

remains the sole support of the posterior inguinal wall.Since the introduction of the term "fascia transversalis" by Sir Ashley Cooper in 1840, this thin layer of tissue has been discovered, denied, and redefined. The transversalis fascia was originally described as a bilaminar membrane. The description he made in 1807 of two laminae has been essentially ignored or denied.Although most subsequent descriptions do not reflect this analysis, some authors, especially in the surgical literature, believe that a posterior lamina of the transversalis fascia exists.

This fascial layer, which is thought to invest the entire abdominal cavity, is a source of controversy for surgeons and anatomists. Some argue that it is a weak layer with no intrinsic strength, while others regard it as essential both in the origin and repair of groin hernias. It is likely that both of these statements are true and almost certainly represent observations from different groups of patients or cadavers. Some regard it as a bilamellar structure with a strong anterior layer and a membranous deep layer[1].

There is little doubt from the laparoscopist's point of view that a two-layer fascial structure exists. The anterior layer of transversalis fascia can be seen easily when reducing a direct hernia as an attenuated fascial structure that lines the defect. The deep layer is observed when entering the pre-peritoneal space subumbilically and immediately posterior to the rectus muscle . Both structures appear strong and difficult to break through in the young patient with an indirect hernia; in older patients, both are flimsy, presumably because of a deficiency of collagen[2].

Some regard the deep layer as a distinct structure from the transversalis fascia. However, as it is followed laterally it appears to interdigitate with the abdominal muscles, making it likely that it is attenuated posterior rectus sheath and will thus contain a fascial contribution from the transversalis fascia[3]. The deep posterior lamina has been confused with a membranous condensation in the preperitoneal fascia.However, Lytle and Fowler reported a secondary or deeper internal ring and Mackay described the inferior epigastric artery perforating the transversalis fascia at its origin and then coursing cephalad on it to enter the rectus sheath anterior to the arcuate line.

It is also likely that the so called anterior layer of transversalis fascia is merely an attenuation of the aponeuroses of the internal oblique and transversus abdominus muscles. Evidence for this comes from children and young adults, in whom this layer is mainly muscular or musculo-tendinous[4].

The transversus abdominus muscle is the deepest of the three abdominal muscle layers and the one seen through the laparoscopic view. It arises from the costal cartilages of the lower six ribs, the vertebral column and the iliac crest. Its fibers run transversely, except in the lower abdomen, where they arch over the inguinal canal as an aponeurotic arch, which is inserted into the pubic crest and iliopectineal line.

The transverse fibers proceed horizontally to their insertion in the rectus sheath and linea Alba. Below the aponeurotic arch, the posterior wall of the inguinal canal is closed by transversalis fascia only in adults and is the site through which direct hernias occur. When the aponeuroses of the transversus and the internal oblique muscle are fused lateral to the rectus sheath, the term 'conjoined tendon' is used. This is a variable structure, however, and does not exist in all patients [5].

Stoppa et al., beginning in **1965**, performed giant prosthetic reinforcement of the visceral sac, covering Fruchaud's myopectineal orifice preperitoneally with extensive overlap.

This is the avascular, fissile, envelope in which Stoppa has so successfully placed prostheses. Preperitoneal approaches to the repair of primary, bilateral, recurrent, inguinal, and femoral herniae, the most common abdominal protrusions, now dominate techniques of repair.He performed much of the innovative work that ultimately formed the foundation for a successful laparoscopic approach to hernia repair. Stoppa's contribution to herniology was that he suggested managing hernias of the groin with a very large, permanent prosthesis that would functionally replace the transversalis fascia[6][7].This experience led to the discovery of the preperitoneal space of Bogros, which, in the 1870 s, was employed for the anterior repair of groin herniation. It is designed in to Retzius and bogros space in the pre peritoneal space and insufflated with carbon dioxide gas, done with a specially designed balloon. This procedure has multifactorial limitations which are individualized with close attention to the complexity and size of the hernia, the patient's comorbidities, and the patient's surgical history.

Rue des Macons described his preperitoneal space which continues into the suprapubic space of Retzius. .

Cheatle demonstrated the median posterior preperitoneal approach, resurrected by Henry .

McEvedy modified the Cheatle-Henry procedure by using a unilateral oblique incision in the rectus sheath and underlying transversalis fascia with medial retraction of the rectus muscle.

Myopectineal orifice

The term **myopectineal orifice** was coined originally by **Dr. Henri Fruchaud**, and refers to a "distinct area of weakness in the pelvic region". The term [**myopectineal**] arises from two **root terms** which are **combined**. The root term [-my-] means "muscle" and the term [-pect-] means "comb"or "**pectinate**". The word [pectineal] in this case refers to the pelvic bone area of origin of the pectinate muscle of the thigh.Fruchaud postulated that the anterior abdominal wall has an area that is inherently weak, and that this area is genetically determined. As such, **hernias** are part of human nature, or as he stated, "a healthy man is, unknown to himself, a hernia bearer".

The orifice as described by **Henri Fruchaud** in 1956 **(Fig-65).**He described the margins of this orifice as follows: lateral boundary as the iliopsoas muscle, medial boundary as rectus sheath and rectus abdominis muscle, superiorly as the arching fibers of transversus abdominis and internal oblique muscle and tendons. He described the inferior boundary of this orifice as the ilio-pectineal line and Cooper's ligament and Pecten pubis.[8][9] The lateral boundary of the orifice is formed by the arching fibers of the internal oblique and transversus abdominis muscle as they arise from the upper surface of the inguinal ligament. The ileopsoas muscle, actually, constitute the postero-laterla boundary of the MPO.

The orifice is subdivided into two regions, femoral below and inguinal above by the inguinal ligament. So, there is a relationship between direct and femoral hernia, one pushing anteriorly and the second one inferiorly[8].

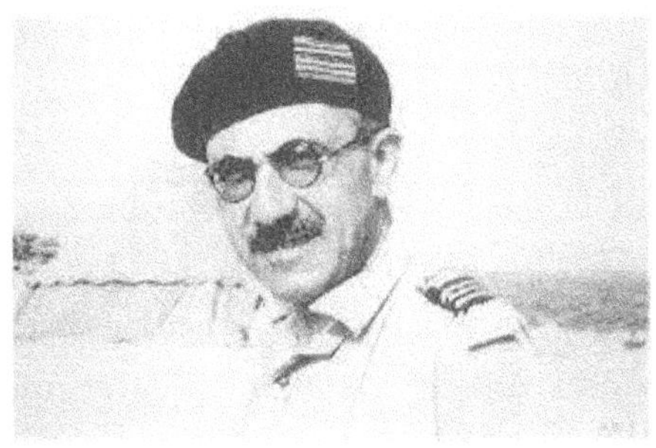

Fig – 65.Henri Fruchaud (1894–1960): A man of bravery, an anatomist a surgeon. Born in 1894 in Angers, the capital of the French province of Anjou.

References

1. Cooper A. The Anatomy and Surgical Treatment of Abdominal Hernia. London: Longman, 1804
2. Wagh PV, Read RC. Collagen deficiency in rectus sheath of patients with inguinal herniation. Proc Soc Exp Biol Med 1971; 37: 382–4.
3. Arregui ME. Surgical anatomy of the preperitoneal fascia and posterior transversalis fascia in the inguinal region. Hernia 1997; 1: 101–10.
4. Bendavid R. The transversalis fascia: new observations in abdominal wall hernias. In: Bendavid R, Abrahamson J,

Arregui ME, et al., eds. Abdominal Wall Hernias: Principles and Management. New York: Springer-Verlag, 2001: 97–100

5. Sorg J, Skandalakis JE, Gray SW. The emperor's new clothes or the myth of the conjoined tendon. Ann Surg 1979; 45: 588–9.
6. Stoppa RE, Petit J, Henry X. Unsutured Dacron prosthesis in groin hernias. Int Surg 1975; 60: 411–15.
7. Stoppa RE, Rives JL, Warlaumont CR, et al. The use of Dacron in the repair of hernias of the groin. Surg Clin N Am 1993; 73: 571–81.
8. Fruchaud H. (1956) Anatomie chirurgicale des hernies de l'aine. Doin, Paris, pp 299-303 and pp 336-342.
9. Wolloscheck T, Konerding MA. Dimensions of the myopectineal orifice: a human cadaver study. Hernia. 2009;13(6):639–642.

9.HISTORY OF ABDOMINAL WALL COMPONENT SEPERATION

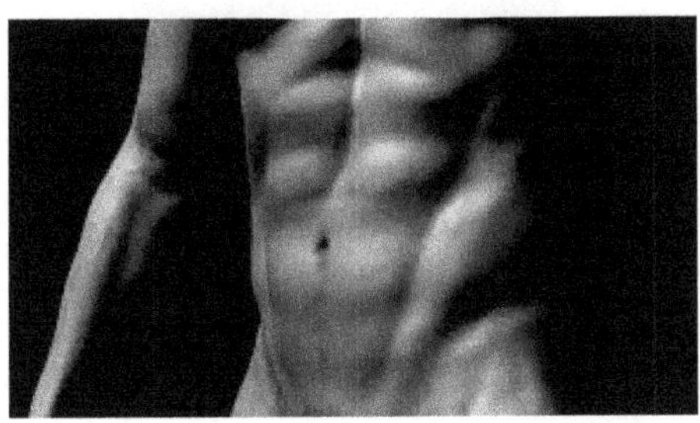

In **1946**, Owen Harding Wangensten (Fig-66) reported the repair of large abdominal defects by pedicled to fascial flaps. In **1983**, Ger and Duboys (Fig -67) described muscle transposition; however, denervation resulted in muscle atrophy and abdominal wall protuberance.

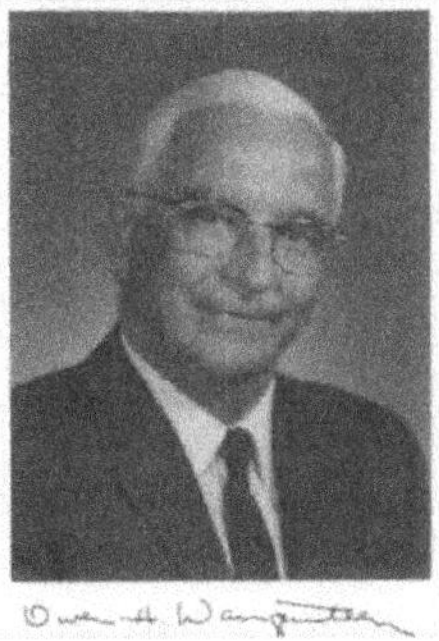

Fig-66.Owen Harding Wangensten Surgeon in chief University of Minnesota Hospitals (1930-1967)

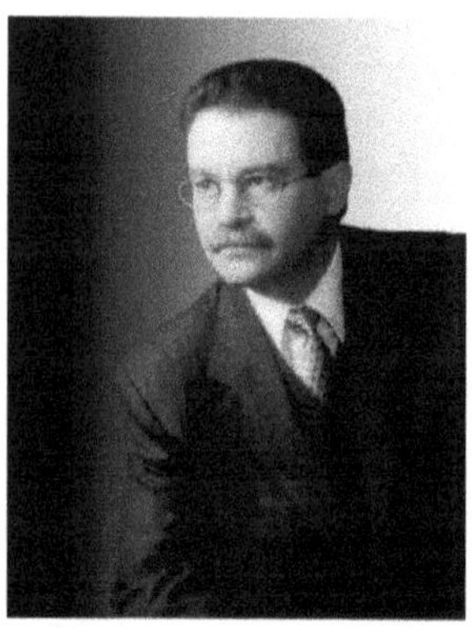

**Fig-67 . , Elliot B Duboys
West Jericho Turnpike
Huntington, NY.**

In 1990, Ramirez *et al.* [1] (Fig- 68) first described the technique of anterior components separation (ACS) to aid in medial fascial advancement and definitive reconstruction. He and his colleagues pioneered the open component separation (OCS) technique. They used bilateral abdominal musculofascial complexes transposed medially to reconstruct ventral abdominal wall defects up to 20 cm at the waistline without the use of prosthetic mesh.

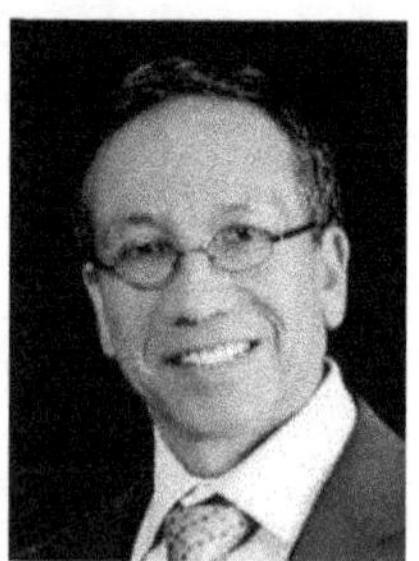

**Fig – 68.Oscar M. Ramirez
Plastic Surgeon, inventor of the "Components Separation Technique".**

This open technique requires the dissection of skin and subcutaneous fatty tissue off the anterior rectus sheath as well as the external oblique aponeurosis.

This allows transaction of the external oblique aponeurosis longitudinally from the costal margin to the level of the inguinal ligament. The external oblique muscle is then separated from the underlying internal oblique muscle. The extensive tissue dissection and undermining not only leads to large seromas and hematomas, but by interrupting the blood supply to the abdominal wall there is an increased rate of tissue ischemia with resultant wound infection and wound dehiscence. Complication rates for open component separation up to 41 percent have been reported.

Saulis and Dumainian (Fig-69) modified the open technique by preserving the peri-umbilical perforating vessels and noted a profound reduction in wound ischemia. However, the dissection still resulted in large hematomas and seromas.

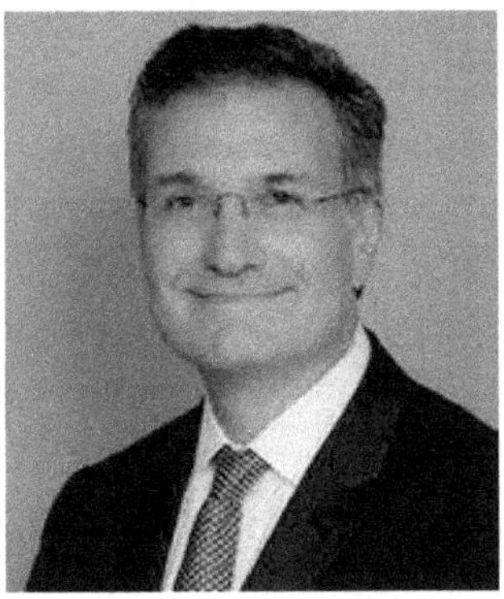

Fig-69.Gregory A Dumanian, Chicago, IL

Another novel technique is the retromuscular (Rives-Stoppa) hernia repair, which was first described in the early 1970s and uses the space between the posterior rectus fascia and the rectus muscle, extending ~6–8 cm on either side of the midline [2][3][4][5][6].

Although durable, the Rives-Stoppa technique is limited by the lateral border of the posterior rectus sheath, and thus usually is inadequate for larger abdominal wall defects. As a result, several modifications on this technique have been developed. Such innovative approaches involve the use of the preperitoneal space or development of an intramuscular plane using a posterior component separation (PCS) technique [7][8].

Another modification of PCS technique, which using transversus abdominis muscle release (TAR) allows significant posterior rectus fascia advancement with preservation of the neurovascular supply, provides a large space for mesh sublay and avoids subcutaneous tissue undermining. Early descriptions by Novitsky and Elliott of the use of TAR starting with a case series of 42 patients undergoing TAR demonstrated a 7.1% wound infection rate and 4.7% recurrence rate with follow-up averaging 26 months. Recurrence rates after components separation have been reported to be 10–22%, with mean follow-up periods ranging from 9.5 months to 4.5 years.

Over time, additional methods of external oblique release have been developed including periumbilical perforator-sparing components separation and endoscopic components separation with the intention of reducing the skin flaps needed to perform this release and thereby preserving the blood supply and minimizing wound morbidity[9][10][11][12] .

Another modification of PCS technique, which using transversus abdominis muscle release (TAR) allows significant posterior rectus fascia advancement with preservation of the neurovascular supply, provides a large space for mesh sublay and avoids subcutaneous tissue undermining [13]. Moreover, TAR technique decreases skin flaps and is usually performed during traditional anterior component release.

Moreover, myofascial advancement during component release was considered as the most physiological reconstruction of large abdominal wall defects as it is based on mobilization and medial advancement of the abdominal wall musculature and accompanying fascia to obliterate the hernia defect using autologous tissue[14]

.

Laparoscopic version of abdominal wall component separation surgery is described in the next chapter.

Referrences

1. Ramirez OM, Ruas E, Dellon AL. 'Components separation' method for closure of abdominal-wall defects: an anatomic and clinical study. Plast Reconstr Surg 1990; 86:519–526.

2. Stoppa RE. The treatment of complicated groin and incisional hernias. World J Surg 1989; 13:545–554.

3. Rives J, Pire JC, Flament JB, Palot JP, Body C. Treatment of large eventrations. New therapeutic

indications apropos of 322 cases. Chirurgie 1985; 111:215–225.

4. Wantz GE. Giant prosthetic reinforcement of the visceral sac. The Stoppa groin hernia repair. Surg Clin North Am 1998; 78:1075–1087.
5. Iqbal CW, Pham TH, Joseph A, Mai J, Thompson GB, Sarr MG. Long-term outcome of 254 complex incisional hernia repairs using the modified rives-Stoppa technique. World J Surg 2007; 31:2398–2404.
6. Mehrabi M, Jangjoo A, Tavoosi H, Kahrom M, Kahrom H. Long-term outcome of rives-Stoppa technique in complex ventral incisional hernia repair. World J Surg 2010; 34:1696–1701.
7. Stoppa R, Petit J, Abourachid H, Henry X, Duclaye C, Monchaux G, Hillebrant JP. Original procedure of groin hernia repair: interposition without fixation of Dacron tulle prosthesis by sub peritoneal median approach. Chirurgie 1973; 99:119–123.
8. Carbonell AM, Cobb WS, Chen SM. Posterior components separation during retro muscular hernia repair. Hernia 2008; 12:359–362.
9. .Harth KC, Rosen MJ. Endoscopic versus open component separation in complex abdominal wall reconstruction. Am J Surg 2010; 199:342–346.
10. Saulis AS, Dumanian GA. Periumbilical rectus abdominis perforator preservation significantly reduces superficial wound complications in 'separation of parts' hernia repairs. Plast Reconstr Surg 2002; 109:2275-2280.
11. Rosen MJ, Williams C, Jin J, McGee MF, Schomisch S, Marks J, Ponsky J. Laparoscopic versus open-component

separation: a comparative analysis in a porcine model. Am J Surg 2007; 194:385–389.

12. Lowe JB, Garza JR, Bowman JL, Rohrich RJ, Strodel WE. Endoscopically assisted 'components separation' for closure of abdominal wall defects. Plast Reconstr Surg 2000; 105:720–729.

13. Novitsky YW, Elliott HL. Transversus abdominis muscle release: a novel approach to posterior component separation during complex abdominal wall reconstruction. Am J Surg 2012; 204:709–716.

14. Breuing K, Butler CE, Ferzoco S, Franz M, Hultman CS, Kilbridge JF *et al.* Incisional ventral hernias: review of the literature and recommendations regarding the grading and technique of repair. Surgery 2010; 148:544–558.

10. HISTORY OF LAPAROSCOPIC HERNIIA

The history of open surgery for hernia is a huge subject and enormous.There are very minute aspects and the inventors of the surgical procedures are available in the big textbooks of the hernia.Iam focusing only on the minimally invasive way of the hderniology in this chapter with the available study material.

Thus, late in the 18th century, surgeons began incising the groin to treat aneurysms there. This experience led to the discovery of the preperitoneal space of Bogros[1], (Bogros **-1786-1825**) described a triangular space in the iliac region between the iliac fascia, transversalis fascia, and parietal peritoneum .The posterior pre-peritoneal approach became established in the 1920s-1960s, along with the use of prostheses.

Laparoscopicrepair of groin protrusions began in **1982**. Potential benefits of the laparoscopic approach include quicker postoperative recovery and possible decreased incidence of long-term groin pain.

With the advent of computer chip technology, laparoscopic visualisation and treatment of inguinal hernia got introduced in the surgical arena. The early **1990's** saw a rapid rise of the number of publications, confirming the feasibility of laparoscopic hernia repair.

The advent of many laparoscopic techniques has made an important number of minimally invasive approaches to inguinal hernia. TAPP technique first published by Lawson Tait [2]in **1891**.

In **1993** the technique of trans-abdominal pre peritoneal (TAPP) has been described based on the same principle of Lawson Tait (Fig – 70) as he described a trans-abdominal approach to the inguinal region performed simultaneously along with other interventions for a laparotomy[3].

In **laparoscopic** TAPP, the same rationale is used and a mesh is placed in the preperitoneal space by incising the peritoneum.

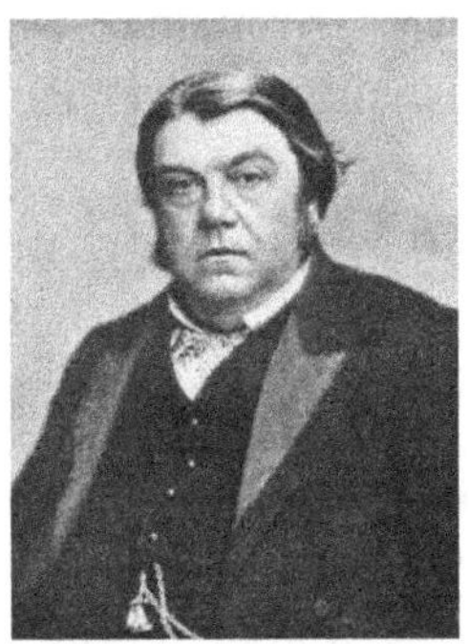

Fig -70 . Lawson Tait, Edinburgh, Scotland, A pioneer in pelvic and abdominal surgery (1845 –1899)

Ger[4] reported the first laparoscopic hernia repair in a paper published in **1982**.This study conducted from August through November **1977** examined the effectiveness of stainless-steel clips to secure the peritoneal opening of known abdominal hernias during laparotomy for other major abdominal procedures. In the thirteenth and final case of the series, an operating laparoscope was used to visualize the peritoneal defect of a right indirect inguinal hernia.

The neck of the hernia sac was closed with a specially devised stapling device passed through a port placed in the right iliac fossa. The staple was constructed of tantalum and measured 12.5 mm long in the open position.

Ger reported that the first patient to be treated by laparoscopic closure of the neck of the sac was under the care of Dr P. Fletcher of the University of the West Indies, Jamaica[4]. Indeed, many surgeons worldwide had immediately started their laparoscopic experience on patients, in contrast to various other techniques in surgical practice, where animal experiments precede evaluation in humans. Moreover in an era where trials were in common use for new drugs, instruments or techniques, trials in laparoscopy on the contrary were performed scarcely and late, and yielded results only years after the already liberal use of laparoscopy.

In **1990**, Popp[5] published a report of the coincidental repair of an inguinal hernia during laparoscopic uterine myomectomy.In this paper, Popp related that the hernia margins were apposed and secured by endosutures tied extracorporeally. A patch of dehydrated dura mater was applied to the sutured area to further cover the repair site.

At the annual meeting of the American Association of Gynecological Laparoscopists (AAGL) in 1989, Bogojavlensky showed a video that demonstrated repair of an indirect inguinal hernia with a laparoscopic stuffing technique[6].The hernia canal was filled with a plug of polypropylene mesh, and the internal ring was closed with suture placed laparoscopically.

In **1990**, Schultz and colleagues reported on a plugand-patch technique for hernia repair that expanded on the initial work described by gynaecologists[7].In 1991, Corbitt independently described a similar technique; however, he further ligated the inverted hernia sac with an endoscopic linear stapler[8].Both Schultz and Corbitt abandoned the technique of plugand-patch repair because of excessive hernia recurrence and changed their technique to one that utilized a large prosthesis of polypropylene mesh in the pre-peritoneal space that covered the entire myopectineal orifice[9].

In **1991**, along with Salerno and colleagues[10],took a somewhat different approach to laparoscopic hernia repair. Both groups reported on an intra-abdominal onlay technique subsequently dubbed the intraperitoneal onlay of mesh (IPOM) procedure[11]. Salerno and colleagues, in an animal model, investigated polypropylene as an onlay prosthesis[12]. Toy and Smoot utilized a prosthesis of expanded polytetrafluoroethylene (ePTFE) stapled to the peritoneal surface. The IPOM procedure was satisfactory for small to moderately sized defects. However, because staple bites were shallow (grasping principally peritoneum) and because of difficulties in visualizing substantial pre-peritoneal structures (Cooper's ligament, iliopubic tract, transversalis fascia, transversus abdominus aponeurosis, etc.), larger hernias repaired with this technique frequently recurred. With increased intra-abdominal pressure, such as with coughing, straining or exercise, the mesh (attached principally to peritoneum) would slide into the hernia defect and the repair would fail.

While the intraabdominal onlay technique was being developed, several groups, led most notably by Arregui [13] and Dion [14], reported on a transabdominal pre-peritoneal patch technique that eventually became adopted widely. In no small measure, this technique relied on the principles of hernia repair established by Stoppa and his GPRVS.

To reduce the potential for complications associated with a peritoneal incision or the intra-abdominal application of a synthetic prosthesis, several authors, including McKernan and Laws[15],Dulucq,[16]and Phillips,[17]discussed a totally extraperitoneal approach to laparoscopic groin hernia repair. This method, which would become known as the total extraperitoneal (TEP) patch procedure, deployed all laparoscopic instrumentation, cannulae, and camera in a working pre-peritoneal space outside of the peritoneal cavity.

In 1993, LeBlanc and Booth described their experience with repair of incisional hernia using ePTFE prosthetic graft[18]. Franklin and colleagues reported on the use of open-weave polypropylene mesh for repair of ventral hernias.[19].Dual-mesh has a rough side and a smooth side. The smooth side of the ePTFE graft is intended to interface with intra-abdominal content and to not excite [20]. Laparoscopic inguinal/femoral hernioplasty adhesion formation.

The rough side is placed in apposition to the abdominal wall, where its rough surface encourages tissue adhesion. The graft is fixed circumferentially with staples or tacks and anchored with transfascial stay sutures placed at the four cardinal points of the graft. Carbajo and colleagues prospectively compared laparoscopic with open prosthetic repair of large incisional hernias [21]. Their study suggested that laparoscopic repair reduces complication rates and hernia recurrence compared with open methods

Beatus Ignatius La Chausse first defined ventral hernia as any hernia that is not inguinal, umbilical, or femoral.The first documented surgery for incisional hernia - Pierre Nicholas Gerdy **(1836)** Completed the surgery by inverting the Hernial sac through the hernia into the abdominal cavity that includes the skin Sutured the edges together and injected ammonia into the sac to cause adhesions.**1910** Kirshner used all types of grafts.Only autologous grafts offered promising results .Loewe (1913) Skin grafts to repair incisional hernias.Nutall (1926) used rectus muscle.Grafts the fascia lata, dura, cartilage, periosteum, and decalcified bone.Synthetic materials introduced in 1940 .Aquaviva, Bonnet, and Maloney used nylon. In **1961** - polypropylene was discovered by Giulio Natta and Karl Ziegler It was popularized for hernia use in **1963** by Francis Usher.He is a general surgeon in Houston, Texas USA with a degree in pharmacology, on the part-time staff of Baylor University and the Veterans Hospital He became interested in plastic prostheses after poor results with dural grafts .He Used custom made polypropylene mesh made out of knitting suture into mesh on animals before applying it on humans .He went on to say that in order to prevent the recurrence mesh needed to be under laid.Burger et al did a comparison between mesh repair and sutured repair showed a recurrence of 32% as compared to 63% for sutured repair during a 6–7-year follow-up. Another approach consisted in making an intraperitoneal U-type incision in the peritoneal wall and inserting the mesh in a preperitoneal position. It became known as the TAPP technique (Trans Abdominal Pre Peritoneal approach).

First laparoscopic ventral hernia repair done by LeBlanc and Booth in **1993** .At present 20% to 27% of repairs are performed laparoscopically .Various aspects have been developed .Transfascial fixation,Tackers (absorbable and non absorbable) or Intracorporeal sutures

In **1989**, the gynaecologist S.Bogojavalensky showed a video demonstrating the laparoscopic intra abdominal incision of the peritoneal hernia sac, subsequently closing the visible muscular defect with a rolled-up piece of polypropylene mesh. A first attempt was made by applying a synthetic mesh to the peritoneal defective wall.

It got the name IPOM (Intra Peritoneal Onlay Mesh). **1991**, Intraperitoneal onlay mesh repair developed by Tay and Smoot, effective for smaller defects.

This was followed by an explosion of laparoscopic procedures, including the first laparoscopic ventral hernia repair done by Leblanc (Fig-71) and Booth[22]described the first laparoscopic ventral hernia repair (LVHR) in 1991. It is based on the same physical and surgical principles as the open underlay procedure described by Stoppa[23],Rives et al[24],and Wantz[25].

LVHR is now being used with increasing frequency, even for the management of complex incisional hernias. Most reports on this topic have supported minimal postoperative morbidity, a shorter convalescence period, and an acceptable recurrence rate[26].

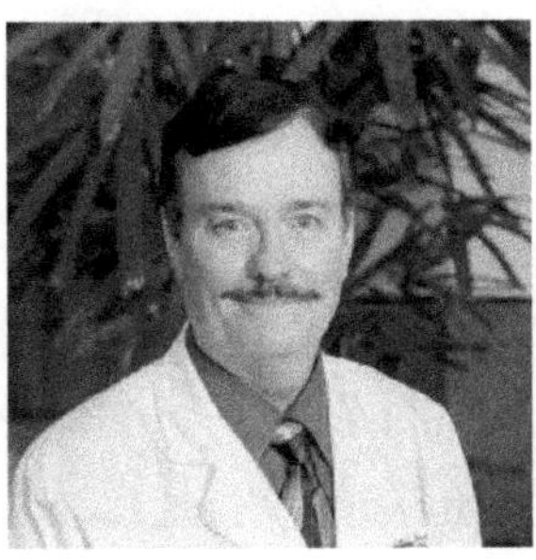

Fig-71.Karl A. LeBlanc, Breaux Bridge, LA

Ventral hernia repair is often culmination of a complex decision-making process by the surgeon. Defect size, location, patient comorbidities, the presence of contamination, acuity of the patient's presentation, necessity for an ostomy, and history of prior repairs with or without a prosthetic all weigh into the ultimate repair approach. The repertoire of operations available does nothing to simplify the matter.

Laparoscopic and open approaches are complicated by innumerable prosthetic choices, and the choice of mesh is next met with a judgment regarding the location of its placement relative to the abdominal wall. Underlay, onlay, inlay, and sublay reinforcement are all viable options that typically compliment the approach. Finally, measurements of success can be equally ambiguous.

In **1992**, Arregui(Fig - 72) et al. and Dion and Morin reported on their transabdominal preperitoneal (TAPP) approach[27] .

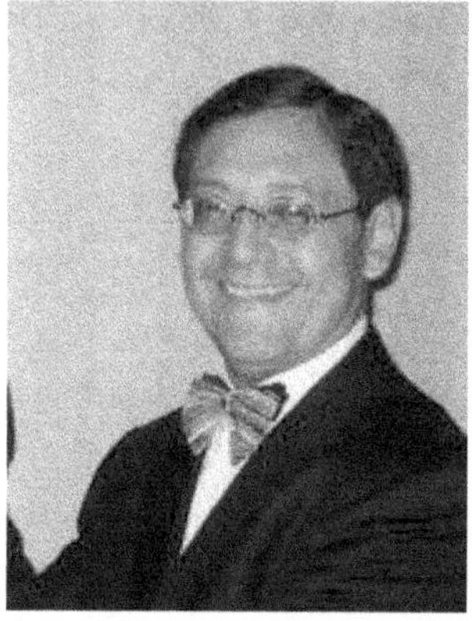

Fig – 72.Maurice E. Arregui, Indianapolis, state of Indiana, U.S.

To avoid intraperitoneal complications, Dulucq recommended a totally extraperitoneal (TEP) approach[28]. Laparoscopic totally extraperitoneal inguinal hernia repair,Lessons learned from 3,100 hernia repairs over 15 years[29].In1993, McKernon and Laws report first totally extraperitoneal (TEP) repair.**January 1993**,Laparoscopic repair of inguinal hernias using a totally extraperitoneal prosthetic approach[30].

These techniques incur fewer recurrences than open techniques and diminish postoperative pain. However, the operating time is longer, they are more expensive, and special skills are needed. In addition, general anaesthesia is required. To avoid intraperitoneal complications, Dulucq (Fig -73) recommended a totally extraperitoneal (TEP) approach.

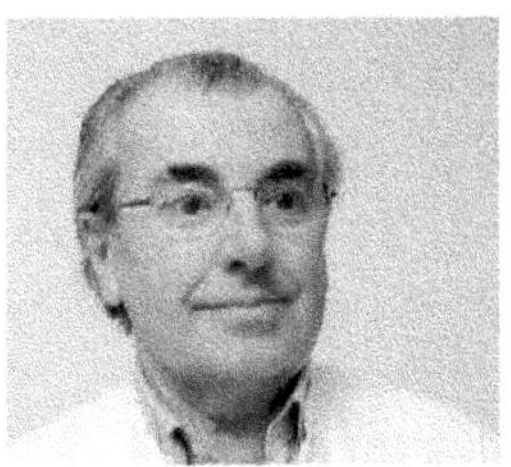

Fig – 73.Jean Luis Dulucq Bordeaux, France

Corbitt modified this technique by inverting the hernia sac and performing a high ligation with sutures or with an endoscopic stapling device used for transection of tissues similar to that used for open bowel resection[31].

When the first trials with often small numbers of patients were published, no real differences in outcome were observed between standard Shouldice or Lichtenstein repairs and laparoscopic techniques. Neither was there at first significant difference between the TAPP and TEP forms of laparoscopic repair. However in all trials reduced pain, as well as earlier ambulation and return to work became strongly apparent. These advantages had to counteract the soon observed higher risk of nerve lesion, resulting in so-called meralgia paresthetica, and the higher financial costs of the use of laparoscopic apparatus. In a later stage, many surgeons favoured the extraperitoneal TEP approach, in view of the absence of adhesion risks in the abdomen.

However, both TAPP and TEP techniques continued to be used in the last 15 years, and are advised as evidence based techniques, equal to Lichtenstein repair. As it stands now, as well open techniques with tension free repair (Lichtenstein repair), as laparoscopic techniques with preperitoneal mesh placement (TAPP or TEP) are the evidence-based and accepted methods in use to deal with adult inguinal hernia. It will be interesting to evaluate how these actual types of hernia repair evolve in the future.

Balloon dissection and telescopic dissection with/ without prior needle insufflation is introduced by Dulucq and recently in **2009**, Edward Felix documented that 'Initially, the dissection of the extraperitoneal space in the TEP approach tended to be difficult, confusing and therefore hard to learn', ratifying the early experience of difficulty and time-consuming nature of the TEP hernioplasty and often time-consuming as well as frustrating.

In **1997**, Lowe et al introduced the concept of using balloon dissectors and endoscopy to facilitate component separation. Around the same time modifications of the technique by Mass et al simplified the endoscopic approach[32].

In **2007**, Rosen (Fig -74) et al improved on the endoscopic technique by successfully avoiding the lengthy subcutaneous undermining with avascular separation of parts[33]. Rosen and colleagues showed that there was no statistically significant difference in the amount of abdominal wall mobilization between ECS and OCS. Open and endoscopic components separation have similar rates of recurrence. The endoscopic group had shorter lengths of stay and less major wound complications[34]. The endoscopic approach may be the ideal technique for complex abdominal wall reconstruction.

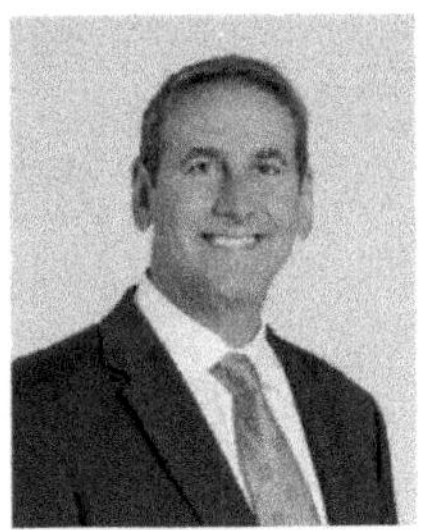

Fig – 74.Michael J Rosen

Professor of Surgery ,Cleveland Clinic Foundation, Cleveland. Ohio.

The arrival of the laparoscopic intra-peritoneal mesh repair in the 1990s with initial attempts at laparoscopically recreating the Rives-Stoppa (RS) repair were technically demanding. Miserez etal. devised an endoscopic, entirely extra-peritoneal approach which did not see wide adoption [35]. It was years later that barbed sutures and the concept of transversus abdominis release were developed, both of which would have eased the surgery considerably.

Extended / Enhanced view of totally extraperitoneal repair (eTEP) is a novel technique that was first introduced by Jorge Daes in 2012 to address difficult inguinal hernias.[36] The principle is to create a larger space than what is done in TEP to tackle large groin hernias.

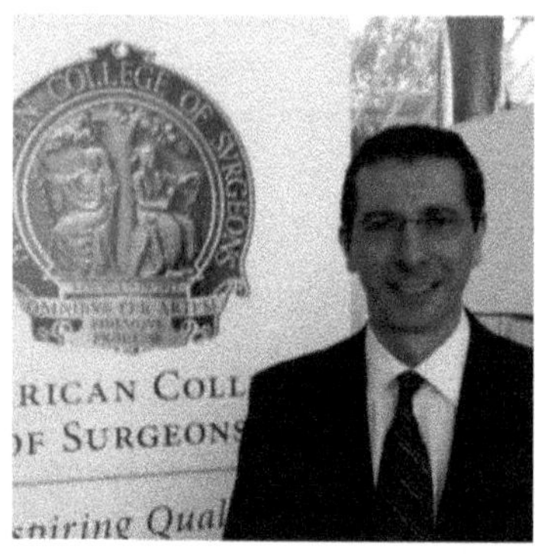

Fig-75.Jorge Daes Daccarett

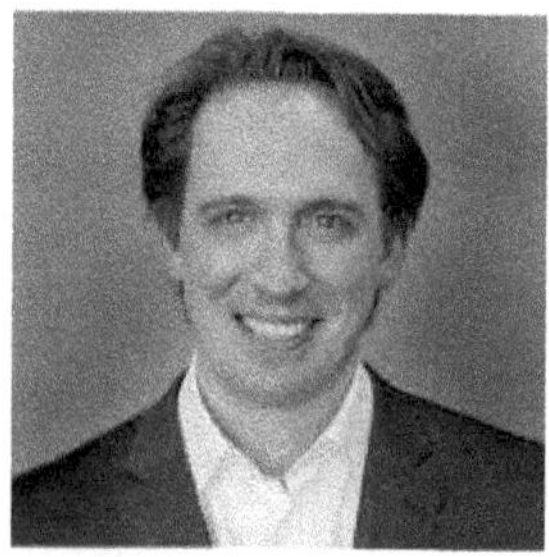

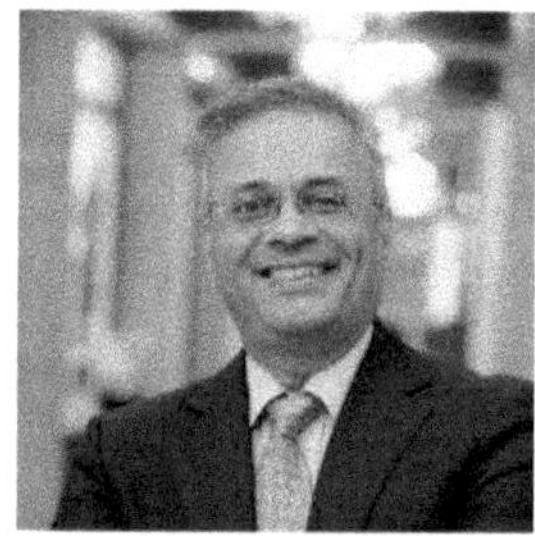

Fig-76. Igor Belyansky Fig 77.Ramana Balasubramaniyan

Works of pioneers such as Dr. Yuri Novitsky, and Dr. Igor Belyansky(Fig-76) have started a new era in the field of hernia surgery. Conventional and popular surgeries for ventral hernias are open onlay mesh hernioplasty, open retromuscular mesh hernioplasty (Rives-Stoppa procedure) and laparoscopic intraperitoneal mesh hernioplasty. Evidence seems to suggest that retromuscular mesh hernioplasty has advantages over other procedures regarding recurrence and surgical site occurrences.

An alternative strategy has been developed for this setting where a mesh is placed in retromuscular space by minimal access technique of the extended Totally

Extraperitoneal approach (eTEP). In 2017, Belyansky et.al. devised the "extended" or "enhanced" view total extra-peritoneal approach (eTEP) for ventral hernias [37]. Their technique was an extension of Daes' work in inguinal hernias where camera access was achieved in a retro-rectus space, dissecting down into the hernia.

Many important signs were described by Balasubramaniyan et.al[38 (Fig - 77)].The "lamppost sign" signals the lateral limit of retro-rectus dissection, preventing iatrogenic injury to the neurovascular bundles and linea semilunaris. After crossover has been safely achieved, the medial edges of the divided posterior rectus sheaths are found connected to each other by a strip of pre-peritoneal fat and peritoneum in the midline. These structures, along with the neck of hernia constitute the "volcano sign". For inferior defects, the vas deferens, the inferior epigastric and gonadal vessels form a triradiate conformation termed the "Mercedes-Benz sign".

Dr. Novitsky is a Professor of Surgery at Columbia University College of Physicians and Surgeons 'known for his expertise in complex inguinal and ventral hernia repairs as well as advanced laparoscopic and robotic surgery. He is perhaps best known for pioneering techniques for abdominal wall reconstructions - the procedure known as transversus abdominis muscle release (TAR). This is called eTEP TAR[39]. It is believed that mesh placement in retromuscular space translates into vascularisation of the mesh from both sides, less recurrence, fewer issues of fixation, less pain and fewer chances of bowel adhesions in addition to being economical due to the deployment of a cheaper mesh as composite mesh with anti-adhesion barrier is not needed[40].

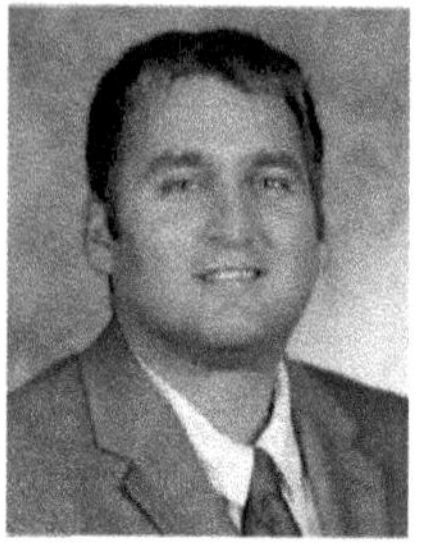

Fig – 78 .Dr. Yuri Novitsky, professor of surgery at University Hospitals Cleveland Medical Centre

References

1. Moments in Surgical History,January 1, 2005,The History of Anatomy and Surgery of the Preperitoneal Space-Petros Mirilas, MD, MSurg; Gene L. Colborn, PhD; David A. McClusky III, MD; et al.
2. Tait L. A discussion on treatment of hernia by median abdominal section. Br Med J 1891;34:685.
3. Litwin DE, Pham QN, Oleniuk FH, Kluftinger AM, Rossi L. Laparoscopic groin hernia surgery: the TAPP procedure. Transabdominal preperitoneal hernia repair. Can J Surg. 1997 Jun;40(3):192-8
4. Ger R. The management of certain abdominal herniae by intra-abdominal closure of the neck of the sac. Ann R Coll Surg Engl 1982; 64: 342–4.
5. Popp LW. Endoscopic patch repair of inguinal hernia in a female patient. Surg Endosc 1990; 4: 10–12
6. Bogojavlensky S. Laparoscopic treatment of inguinal and femoral hernia. Video presentation presented at the 18th Annual Meeting of the American Association of Gynecological Laparoscopists, Washington, DC, 1989.

7. Schultz L, Graber J, Pietrafitta J, Hickok D. Laser laparoscopic herniorrhaphy: a clinical trial preliminary results. J Laparoendosc Surg 1990; 1: 23–5.

8. Corbitt JD. Laparoscopic herniorrhaphy. Surg Laparosc Endosc 1991; 1: 23–5

9. Toy and Smoot42 Toy FK, Smoot RT, Jr. Toy-Smoot laparoscopic hernioplasty. Surg Laparosc Endosc 1991; 1: 151–6.

10. Salerno GM, Fitzgibbons RJ, Filipi C. Laparoscopic inguinal hernia repair. In: Zucker KA, ed. Surgical Laparoscopy. St Louis: Quality Medical Publishing, 1991: 281–93.

11. Fitzgibbons RJ. Laparoscopic inguinal hernia repair. New Frontiers in Endoscopy, Nationwide Satellite Teleconference, May 1991.

12. Salerno GM, Fitzgibbons RJ, Filipi C. Laparoscopic inguinal hernia repair. In: Zucker KA, ed. Surgical Laparoscopy. St Louis: Quality Medical Publishing, 1991: 281–93

13. Arregui ME, Davis CD, Yucel O, et al. Laparoscopic mesh repair of inguinal hernia using a preperitoneal approach: a preliminary report. Surg Laparosc Endosc 1992; 2: 53–8

14. Dion YM, Morin J. Laparoscopic inguinal herniorrhaphy. Can J Surg 1992; 35: 209–12.

15. McKernan BJ, Laws HL. Laparoscopic preperitoneal prosthetic repair of inguinal hernias. Surg Rounds 1992; 7: 579–610.

16. Dulucq JL. Traitement des hernies de l'aine par mise en place d'un patch prothétique sous-péritonéal en rétropéritonéoscopie. Cahiers Chir 1991; 79: 15–16.

17. Phillips EH, Carroll BJ, Fallas MJ. Laparoscopic preperitoneal inguinal hernia repair without peritoneal incision. Surg Endosc 1993; 7: 159–62.

18. LeBlanc KA, Booth WV. Laparoscopic repair of incisional abdominal hernias using expanded polytetrafluoroethylene: preliminary findings. Surg Laparosc Endosc 1993; 3: 39–41.

19. Franklin ME, Heniford BT, Arca MJ, et al. Laparoscopic ventral and incisional hernia repair. Surg Laparosc Endosc 1998; 8: 294–9.

20. Popp LW. Endoscopic patch repair of inguinal hernia in a female patient. Surg Endosc 1990; 4: 10–12

21. Carbajo MA, Martin del Olmo JC, Blanco JI, et al. Laparoscopic treatment vs. open surgery in the solution of major incisional and abdominal wall hernias with mesh. Surg Endosc 1999; 13: 250–2.

22. Leblanc KA, Booth WV. Laparoscopic repair of incisional abdominal hernias using polytetrafluoroethylene: preliminary findings. *Surg Laparosc Endosc*. 1993;3:39–41.

23. .Stoppa RE. The treatment of complicated groin and incisional hernias. *World J Surg*. 1989;13:545–554.

24. Rives J, Pire JC, Flament JB, et al. Treatment of large eventrations: new therapeutic indications apropos of 322 cases. *Chirurgie*. 1985;111:215–225.

25. Wantz GE. Incisional hernioplasty with Mersilene. *Surg Gynecol Obstetr*. 1991;172:129–137.

26. Heniford BT, Park A, Ramshaw BJ, Voeller G. Laparoscopic ventral and incisional hernia repair in 407 patients. *J Am Coll Surg*. 2000;190:645–650.

27. Surg Laparosc Endosc 2:53-58, 1992.

28. Cahiers Chir 79:15-16, 1991.

29. October 2008,Surgical Endoscopy 23(3):482-6

30. J. Barry McKernan & Henry L. Laws -Surgical Endoscopy volume 7, pages26–28 (1993).

31. Corbitt J. Laparoscopic herniorrhaphy. Surg Laparosc Endosc 1991; 1: 23–5

32. Lowe JB, Garza JR, Bowman JL, Rohrich RJ, Strodel WE (2000) Endoscopically assisted "components separation" for

closure of abdominal wall defects. Plast Reconstr Surg 105(2):720–729

33. Am J Surg,2010 Mar;199(3):342-6; discussion 346-7.

34. Rosen MJ, Williams C, Jin J, McGee MF, Schomisch S, Marks J, Ponsky J (2007) Laparoscopic versus open-component separation: a comparative analysis in a porcine model. Am J Surg 194:385–389.

35. Miserez M, Penninckx F (2002) Endoscopic totally preperitoneal ventral hernia repair: surgical technique and short-term results. Surg Endosc Other Interv Tech 16:1207–1213.

36. Daes J. The enhanced view-totally extraperitoneal technique for repair of inguinal hernia. *Surg Endosc.* 2012;26:1187–9.

37. .Belyansky I, Daes J, Radu VG, Balasubramanian R, Reza Zahiri ,H, Weltz AS, Sibia US, Park A, Novitsky Y (2018) A novel approach using the enhanced-view totally extraperitoneal (eTEP) technique for laparoscopic retromuscular hernia repair. Surg Endosc Other Interv Tech 32:1525–1532

38. Signs and landmarks in eTEP Rives-Stoppa repair of ventral hernias, B. Ramana, E. Arora & I. Belyansky Hernia volume 25, pages545–550 (2021).

39. Belyansky I, Daes J, Radu VG, Balasubramanian R, Reza Zahiri H, Weltz AS, et al. A novel approach using the enhanced-view totally extraperitoneal (eTEP) technique for laparoscopic retromuscular hernia repair. *Surg Endosc.* 2018;32:1525–32.

40. Binnebösel M, Klink CD, Otto J, Conze J, Jansen PL, Anurov M, et al. Impact of mesh positioning on foreign body reaction and collagenous ingrowth in a rabbit model of open incisional hernia repair. *Hernia.* 2010;14:71–7.

11. POPULAR NEW TECHNIQUES

SCOLA

Recently this procedure was described by "exclusive" endoscopic technique, that is, through small suprapubic incisions for the portals and CO2 insufflation to maintain the operative field[1][2] .However, this article presents some technical modifications in relation to the original study published by Argentine surgeons, mainly the placement of a larger screen in a pre-aponeurotic position and absence of relaxation incisions, a technique we call SCOLA (Subcutaneous onlay laparoscopic approach)

ELAR

Another alternative is endoscopic-assisted reconstruction of the linea alba, known among others as ELAR (Endoscopic assisted linea alba reconstruction) [3].

It is a hybrid technique that, from a peri-umbilical incision with extension 2-3 cm higher and endoscopic vision aid, the pre-aponeurotic space is dissected until the xiphoid and after, plasturing the diastasis reinforced by the placement of polypropylene mesh (ELAR plus). Several authors have reported satisfactory results with this technique, despite complications related to operative wound in up to 6.4% [4].

MILOS

Alternatives to the pre-aponeurotic techniques have been described and have as main advantage to minimize the incidence of the seroma. Schwarz et al[5] described a hybrid technique that, through a peri-umbilical incision with the aid of endoscopic vision, has the retromuscular space dissected for placement of the mesh, known as MILOS(Mini/less open sublay technique) . Daes et al [6] and Belyansky et al [7] have described and have used totally extraperitoneal techniques for the correction of anterior wall hernias associated with DMRA. Despite very encouraging results, these procedures are more complex and require greater anatomical knowledge and laparoscopic skills than onlay techniques.

In hybrid technique, the mesh is placed laparoscopically. The closure of defects, removal of sac and necrotic skin may be done by open approach. Combining steps of open and laparoscopic techniques is employed to achieve good hernia mesh repair with minimal access and less morbidity. Studies suggest that the hybrid technique is safe in cases of recurrent difficult incisional hernias.[8] Some reports also suggest using hybrid technique for obese patients with difficult incisional hernias, multiple defects, irreducible hernias with necrotic skin, lateral incisional hernias[9] and parastomal hernias.[10].

Referrences

1.Bellido Luque J Bellido Luque A, Valdivia J, Suarez Gráu JM, Gomez Menchero J, García Moreno J, Guadalajara Jurado J. Totally endoscopic surgery on diastasis recti associated with midline hernias The advantages of a minimally invasive approach. Prospective cohort study. *Hernia.* 2015;19(3):493–501.

2. Muas DMJ, Verasay GF, Garcia WM. Reparacio´n endosco´pica prefascial de la dia´stasis de los rectos descripcio´n de una nueva te´cnica. *Rev Hispanoam Hernia.* 2017;5(2):47–51.

3. Köckerling F, Botsinis MD, Rohde C, Reinpold W, Schug-Pass C. Endoscopic-assisted linea alba reconstruction New technique for treatment of symptomatic umbilical, trocar, and/or epigastric hernias with concomitant rectus abdominis diastasis. *Eur Surg.* 2017;49(2):71–75.

4.Köckerling F, Botsinis MD, Rohde C, Reinpold W. Endoscopic-Assisted Linea Alba Reconstruction plus Mesh Augmentation for Treatment of Umbilical and/or Epigastric Hernias and Rectus Abdominis Diastasis - Early Results. *Front Surg.* 2016;3:27–27. doi: 10.3389/fsurg.2016.00027.

5. Schwarz J, Reinpold W, Bittner R. Endoscopic mini/less open sublay technique (EMILOS)-a new technique for ventral hernia repair. Langenbecks Arch Surg. 2017;402(1):173–180. doi: 10.1007/s00423-016-1522-0.

6. Daes J. Endoscopic subcutaneous approach to component separation. *J Am Coll Surg.* 2014;218(1):e1–e4.

7. Belyansky I, Daes J, Radu VG, Balasubramanian R, Reza Zahiri H, Weltz AS, Sibia US, Park A, Novitsky Y. A novel approach using the enhanced-view totally extraperitoneal (eTEP) technique for laparoscopic retromuscular hernia repair.

8. Griniatsos J, Yiannakopoulou E, Tsechpenakis A, Tsigris C, Diamantis T. A hybrid technique for recurrent incisional hernia repair. Surg Laparosc Endosc Percutan Tech 2009;19:e177-80.

9. Schwab R, Sahm J, Willms AG. Video-assisted mini-open sublay (VAMOS): A simple hybrid approach for lateral incisional hernias. Front Surg 2018;5:29.

10. Luo W, Wang Y, Duan X. Therapeutic effect of a new hybrid technique which combined laparoscopic method and abdominal repair for parastomal hernia repair. Zhonghua Wai Ke Za Zhi 2017;55:539-42.

12. Conclusions

1. It is true that endoscopy /laproscopy has struggled a lot in thousands of years.It's the contribution of many physicians and surgeons over many decades of the difficult situations at their working conditions made many innovations for the future generations.
2. It was the journry of making new instruments and inventions by the way of self-experiments on themselves have changed the way of interviening the endoscopic procedures towards the edge of comfirtability and good results.
3. It's not in a single day or years ,these quintessential finest changes got modified in the history of laparoscopy and hernia in which it's appreciated by the below pictures.The reflected light source which was used to view the interior of a human body is evoluted to the level of remotely performing the robotic surgery with the help of finest instruments and technology.

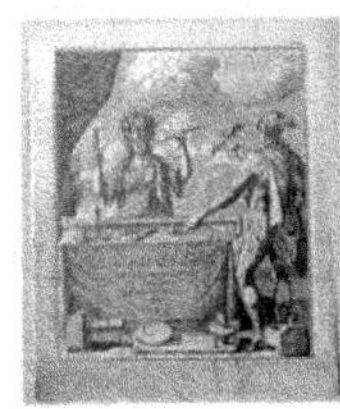

Text Book -The First Optical Instruments as Allegorical Depiction

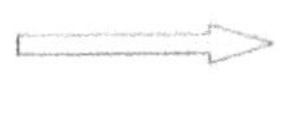

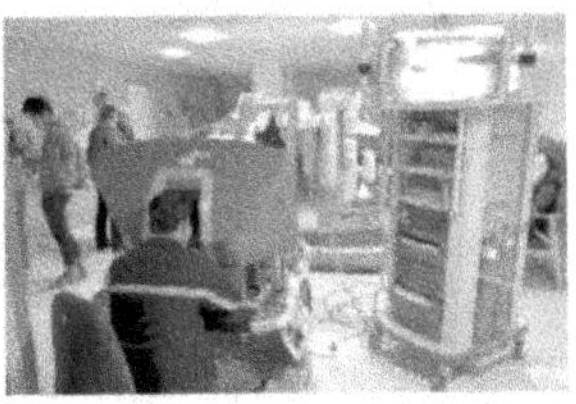

Robotic Surgery

4. The strong innovarive patheway of laparoscopy/endoscopy in each specialities have established their mark of recognition in the clinical trials and studies so that, fresh guidelines and recommendations on a specific surgical procedure are possible now,

5. The futue and growth of endoscopy/minimally invasive surgeries appears promising with new ideas of overcoming the present difficulties with ease if the trend of the nano technology, robotic and artificial intelligence grows parallel to the needs of the people and the performing doctors including with"telepresence surgery".

6. Let us hope that this will not lead to total absence of a human relationship in the surgical operation". Nevertheless, not all the surgeons accepted this revolution, above all among those who were older, and a group formed whose motto was, "Why peek through a key hole when you can open the door?" To which the advocates of laparoscopy responded: "Why kick in the door, when you can look through the key hole?" **(Nord HJ. Laparoscopy- a historical perspective: are gastroenterologists going to reclaim it? Gastrointest Endosc 2008;68:67-68.)**

7. Finally, if the "Ethics" in the practice is focused on the modern laparoscopic and endoscopic procedures, they are riddled with ethical questions like, is it certain that minimal access procedures should be performed on the patients? What are the safety standards? Should society have been using and advocating the technology as it progressed?

8. Is it true that the only way of progression of the science can occur through trial and error but would it have been considered too risky to use on humans? These are the common questions throughout history by many critics who often held the advancements back.

Revolution of minimal access Surgery in India

1.**Dr.Tempton Udwadia** of Hinduja Hospital, Mumbai is accepted by most as the father of Laparoscopic Surgery in India . Two aspects need strong emphasis as he mentioned in **J Minim Access Surg. 2005 Jun; 1(2): 51–52.**

1. Laparoscopic surgery is not a super speciality–it is merely the logical progress of general surgery brought about by advanced technology in instrumentation and imaging. To make this advance available to the entire Indian community irrespective of socio-economic status, it is imperative to spread this advance to every surgeon in India - a goal which can only be achieved if EVERY teaching hospital imparts training in MAS to every resident and EVERY University incorporates this advance as an essential element in its curriculum. As important as spreading this surgery to every surgeon is the necessity to tailor the cost of this surgery by improvisation, to try and give the benefit of this surgery to all our people. This is the real challenge faced by surgeons in India, to realize that laparoscopic surgery can grow in India not with robots but with basic equipment, to go beyond merely following the developed world by devising technology compatible with our country.

2. That a procedure can be done by laparoscopy is not adequate indication to do so. Every laparoscopic procedure must be evaluated and appraised not merely on its feasibility nor by the enthusiasm or euphoria of personal ego or achievement, but rather as a pragmatic clinical study as it applies to our own country and conditions. The history of surgery is replete with many surgical procedures practiced ardently over several decades which subsequently fell by the wayside. Time and an adequate honest follow-up alone will tell us which procedure enters the register of established and accepted practice.

Having said all this, there can be no doubt that MAS is the most compelling and dynamic force driving surgical progress and endeavour in the current era.

2.Dr.Chinnusamy Palanivelu of GEMS Hospital Coimbatore, established CIGES(Coimbatore Institute of Gastrointestinal Endosurgery) in 1991, developed many advances in laparoscopic surgery and contributed significantly to the growth of Minimal Access Surgery in Southern India around the same time. His work on the pancreas has been appreciated and recognized internationally. Along with more than his 239 Publications of various minimal access procedures of surgical gastro enterology and hernia surgeries, his role as a mentor and path director to many surgeons of india is enormous and widely accepted.He is considered as the father of laparoscopy in south and north india with world wide participation and recognition as a first one who performed a laparoscopic Whipple's surgery for cancer in 2007.His innovations and teaching programmes are everlasting to the next generation surgeons who are always in zeal of learning minimally invasive surgeries with the practical mode of updates in this competitive world.

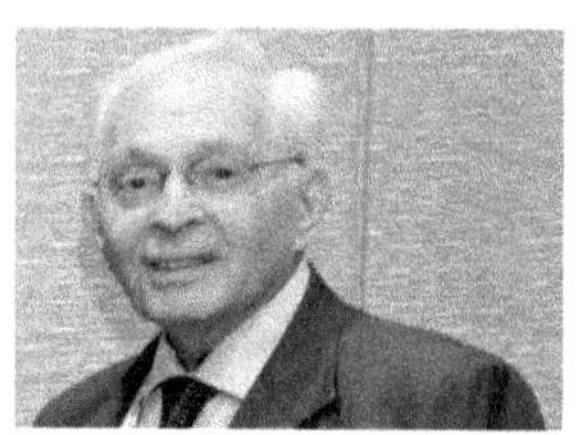

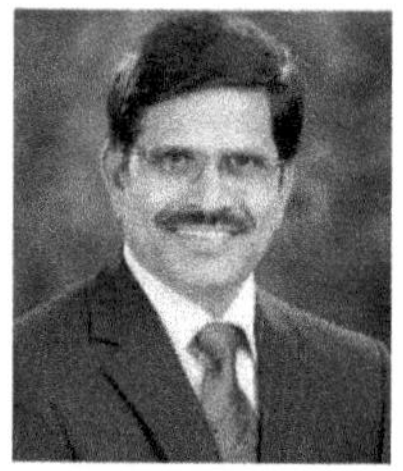

1. Dr.Tempton Udwadia 2. **Dr.Chinnusamy Palanivelu**

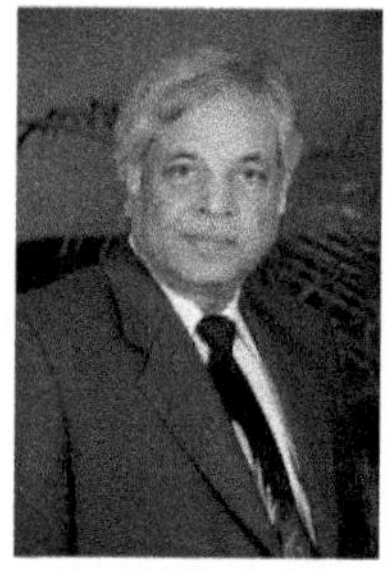

3.**Dr.Pradeep Kumar Chowbey** is a world reknowned laparoscopic and bariatric surgeon,teacher to the surgeons of india and abroad in minimal access surgery and metabolic surgery from max care healthcare institute New Delhi .The Governament of India awarded him the forth highest civilian honour of the Padma Shri in 2002.Besides his more than 158 national and internal publications in Minimally invasive surgery,more than 17 chapters in the textbooks and many awards and records,he is a founding designee in the International Centre of Excellence for Bariatric Surgery Program by Surgical Review Corporation, USA.His contribution to the laparoscopic training and being a mentor in the population of younger generation surgeons in india has remarkably made a stong impact to upgrade in their surgical career.

Reference Text Books

1.History of laparoscopy.,Kaiser AM, Corman ML,Surg Oncol Clin N Am. 2001 Jul

2. G Chir Vol. 33 - n. 3 - pp. 53-57 March 2012.A brief history of laparoscopy

3 .Nezhat C. Nezhat's history of endoscopy: a historical analysis of endoscopy's ascension since antiquity. Tuttlingen: Endo Press; 2011. pp. 1–199.

4.Gotz F, Pier A, Schippers E, Schumpelick V. The history of laparoscopy. In: Gotz F, Pier A, Schippers E, Schumpe- lick V, editors. Color Atlas of Laparoscopic Surgery. New York 1993:3-5.

5. Nezhat C. Nezhat's history of endoscopy: a historical analysis of endoscopy's ascension since antiquity. Tuttlingen: Endo Press; 2011. Pp. 1–199.

6. Edmonson JM. History of the instruments for gastrointestinal endoscopy. Gastrointest Endosc 1991 Mar-Apr; 37(Suppl 2):827-856.

7. G Chir Vol. 33 - n. 3 - pp. 53-57 March 2012.A brief history of laparoscopy

8. Felix EL (2009) Laparoscopic Inguinal Hernia Repair. In: Nathaniel J. Soper, Lee L. Swanstrom, W. Stephen Eubanks (eds.). Mastery of Endoscopic and Laparoscopic Surgery, 3rd Edition, Chapter 53, Philadelphia: Lippincott Williams & Wilkins, pp: 523-537.

9.Belt AE, Charnock DA. The cystoscope and its use. In: Cabot H, editor. Modern urology. Philadelphia (PA): Lea & Febiger; 1936. p. 15-50.

10.Gorden A. The history and development of endoscopic surgery. In: Sutton C, Diamond MP, editors. Endoscopic Sur- gery for Gynecologists. London 1993;3-7.

11. 4.Gunning JE. The history of laparoscopy. J Reprod Med 1974

12. Schollmeyer T, Soyinka AS, Schollmeyer M, et al. Georg Kelling (1866-1945): The root of modern day minimal invasive surgery. A forgotten legend? Arch Gynecol Obstet. 2007;276(5):505-509.

13. Bozzini PH. Lichtleiter. Eine Erfindung zur Anschauung innerer Teile und Krankheiten. J Prak Heilk 1806;24:107-109.

14. Belt AE, Charnock DA. The cystoscope and its use. In: Cabot H, editor. Modern urology. Philadelphia (PA): Lea & Febiger; 1936. P. 15-50.

15.Davis CJ, Filipi JC. A history of endoscopic surgery. In: Arregui ME, Fitzgibbons RJJ, Katkhouda N, McKernan JB, Reich H, editors. Principles of laparoscopic surgery – basic and advanced techniques. New York (NY): Springer-Verlag. p. 3-20.

16. Aranzi GC: Hippocratis librum de vulneribus capitis commentarius cum Claudii Porralii annotationibus marginalibus MDC XXXIX. (Courtesy Austrian Literature Online, Graz University Library, Graz, Austria)

17.Nitze M. Eine neue Beobachtungs- und Untersuchungsmethode für Harnröhre, Harnblase und Rektum. Wien. Med Wschr 1879;29:649-652.

18.Berci G. History of Endoscopy. In: Berci G, editor. Endoscopy. Appleton-Century-Crofts 1976:19-33.

19.Kelling G: Über die Oesophagoskopie, Gastroskopie und Koelioskopie. Münch Med Wschr 1902;49:21-24.

20. Hopkins HH. The modern urological endoscope. In: Gow JG, Hopkins HH, editors. Handbook of urological endoscopy. Edinburgh: Churchill Livingstone; 1978. p. 20-33.

21.William P. Didusch Center for Urologic History, American Urological Association, Linthicum, MD, USA.

22.Von Ott, DO.: Ventroscopic illumination of the abdominal cavity in pregnancy. Akrestierstova Zh, Zhenskikh I Bo- loznei 1901;15:7-10.

23.Marlow J. History of laparoscopy, optics, fiber optics, and instrumentation. Clin Obstet Gynecol 1976 Jun;19(2):261-275.

24.Stein A, Stewart WH. Roentgen examination of the abdominal organs following oxygen inflation of peritoneal cavity. Ann Surg. 1919;70(1):95-100.

25.Jacobaeus HC. Kurze Übersicht über meine Erfahrungen mit der Laparoskopie. Münch Med Wschr 1911;58:2017-2021.

26.Alexander G, Emma J. Laparoscopic surgery historical perspectives In: Zucker K, editor. Surgical laparoscopy. Philadelphia (PA): Lippincott Williams and Wilkins; 2001. p. 3-11.

27.Bernkeim HBM. Organoscopy: ystoscopy of the abdominal cavity. Ann Surg 1911;53:764-767.

28. Litynski GS. Laparoscopy between the World Wars: The barriers to trans-Atlantic exchange. Spotlighting Heinz Kalk and John C. Ruddock. JSLS. 1997;1(2):185-188.

29.Semm K. Atlas of gynecologic laparoscopy and hysteroscopy. Philadelphia (PA): WB Saunders; 1977. P. 7-14.

30.Goetz O. Ein neues Verfahren zur Gasfüllung für das Pneumoperitoneum. Münch Med Wschr 1921;51:233-236.

31.Veress J. Neues Instrument zur Ausfuhrung von Brustoder Bauchpunktionen und Pheumothoraxbehandlung. Deutsche Med Wochenschr 1938;64:1480-1481.

32.Hopkins HH. The modern urological endoscope. In: Gow JG, Hopkins HH, editors. Handbook of urological endoscopy. Edinburgh: Churchill Livingstone; 1978. p. 20-33.

33.Alexander G, Emma J. Laparoscopic surgery historical perspectives In: Zucker K, editor. Surgical laparoscopy. Philadelphia (PA): Lippincott Williams and Wilkins; 2001. P. 3-11.

34.Berci G. History of Endoscopy. In: Berci G, editor. Endoscopy. Appleton-Century-Crofts 1976:19-33.

35.Davis CJ. A history of Endoscopic Surgery. Surg Laparosc Endosc 1992;7:369-373.

www.ingramcontent.com/pod-product-compliance
Ingram Content Group UK Ltd.
Pitfield, Milton Keynes, MK11 3LW, UK
UKHW021649190726
13853UKWH00001B/153

9 789354 724282